Understanding Mesothelioma

This practical text highlights the lived experience of mesothelioma. Following the patient journey and underpinned by the evidence, it explores what good care for mesothelioma looks like. Mesothelioma is complex in its aetiology, presentation, symptom burden and patient pathway. The public health context is shifting, as the way people are exposed to asbestos changes and there are new life-lengthening treatments available with many benefits but also challenges.

This timely book provides the context for mesothelioma, what it is and why it occurs before profiling a range of experiences across the patient pathway to highlight implications for care delivered by nurses and other health and social care practitioners. The second section of the book follows the patient pathway from diagnosis through to end-of-life care and bereavement, highlighting the lived experience and summarising the implications for practice. The final section of the book discusses aspects of the mesothelioma experience that are unique to the condition, including mental health impacts, and financial and legal implications.

Presenting insights that will inform practice in a diverse range of fields, including health, social care and law, this book is an essential reference for all those working with people with mesothelioma and their families. It is also an important reference for those working in cancer care more generally and academics with an interest in the lived experience of health conditions.

Angela Tod is Professor of Older People and Care at the University of Sheffield, UK, and Co-Director of the Mesothelioma UK Research Centre (MURC).

Bethany Taylor is a Research Fellow at the Mesothelioma UK Research Centre (MURC), University of Sheffield, UK.

Clare Gardiner is Professor of Palliative Care at the University of Sheffield, UK, and Co-Director of the Mesothelioma UK Research Centre (MURC).

Liz Darlison is the CEO of Mesothelioma UK and a Nurse Consultant in Mesothelioma.

"This insightful book challenges preconceptions around mesothelioma, revealing the unique adversities faced by patients and carers living with the disease, alongside the expert support provided by clinical nurse specialists. It draws on contemporary evidence of poignant lived experiences, providing an invaluable guide for clinicians supporting patients throughout the mesothelioma journey. An exceptional resource for nursing, medical and allied health professionals."

– **Dr Rachel King**, *University of Sheffield*

"This textbook is an essential resource for anyone involved in the care or research involving patients with mesothelioma. By centring the experiences of patients and their families, it fills a critical gap in the literature. Combining expert insights, international research, and a practice-based approach, it offers invaluable guidance for healthcare professionals navigating this complex disease. Timely and comprehensive, this book is a vital tool for improving care and outcomes for those affected by mesothelioma."

– **Professor Dean Fennell**, *Chair of Thoracic Oncology, University of Leicester*

Understanding Mesothelioma

The Experiences and Care Needs of People with Mesothelioma and their Families

EDITED BY ANGELA TOD,
BETHANY TAYLOR,
CLARE GARDINER AND
LIZ DARLISON

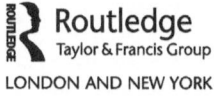

Routledge
Taylor & Francis Group

LONDON AND NEW YORK

Designed cover image: Getty Images

First published 2026
by Routledge
4 Park Square, Milton Park, Abingdon, Oxon OX14 4RN

and by Routledge
605 Third Avenue, New York, NY 10158

Routledge is an imprint of the Taylor & Francis Group, an informa business

British Library Cataloguing-in-Publication Data
A catalogue record for this book is available from the British Library

ISBN: 978-1-032-63130-1 (hbk)
ISBN: 978-1-032-63129-5 (pbk)
ISBN: 978-1-032-63131-8 (ebk)

DOI: 10.4324/9781032631318

Typeset in Vectora LT Std
by KnowledgeWorks Global Ltd.

This book is dedicated to all those past, present and future who have lived with mesothelioma.

Contents

List of contributors ix
Preface xi
Acknowledgements xiii
Glossary xv

1 **Introduction** 1
ANGELA TOD AND CLARE GARDINER

2 **Mesothelioma** 7
LEAH TAYLOR, PETER ALLMARK AND ANGELA TOD

3 **The role of the specialist nurse in multidisciplinary and partnership working** 21
LEAH TAYLOR, SARAH HARGREAVES AND ANGELA TOD

4 **The road to diagnosis** 33
BETHANY TAYLOR AND ANGELA TOD

5 **Treatment experiences** 45
ANNA BIBBY, ANNA MORLEY AND CLARE WARNOCK

6 **Symptoms and their management** 57
DONNA WAKEFIELD, RACHEL SMITHERS AND ANNA BIBBY

7 **The supportive care needs of people with mesothelioma** 69
ZOE DAVEY AND CATHERINE HENSHALL

8 **Clinical trials** 79
BETHANY TAYLOR, LEAH TAYLOR, ANGELA TOD AND SIMON BOLTON

9   Palliative and end-of-life care in mesothelioma   91
    CLARE GARDINER AND SARAH HARGREAVES

10 The legacy of the illness for the family   102
    SARAH HARGREAVES, SARAH THOMAS AND SAMANTHA COX

11 The role of primary care in mesothelioma   114
    EMILIE COUCHMAN

12 Mental health and mesothelioma   125
    VIRGINIA SHERBORNE AND STEPHANIE EJEGI-MEMEH

13 Financial implications   137
    SARAH THOMAS

14 Seeking compensation   149
    JENNIFER SEAVOR

15 Conclusion   162
    ANGELA TOD, CLARE GARDINER, BETHANY TAYLOR AND LIZ DARLISON

Index   165

List of contributors

Peter Allmark, University of Sheffield, UK

Anna Bibby, University of Bristol, UK

Simon Bolton, Mesothelioma UK, UK

Emilie Couchman, University of Sheffield, UK

Samantha Cox, Readley Asbestos and Mesothelioma Support, UK

Zoe Davey, Oxford Brookes University, UK

Stephanie Ejegi-Memeh, University of Sheffield, UK

Sarah Hargreaves, University of Sheffield, UK

Catherine Henshall, Oxford Brookes University, UK

Anna Morley, Mesothelioma UK

Jennifer Seavor, RWK Goodman, UK

Virginia Sherborne, University of Sheffield, UK

Rachel Smithers, North Bristol NHS Trust, UK

Leah Taylor, Mesothelioma UK

Sarah Thomas, Mesothelioma UK

Donna Wakefield, North Tees and Hartlepool NHS Foundation Trust, UK

Clare Warnock, Sheffield Teaching Hospitals NHS Foundation Trust, UK

Preface

Mesothelioma is a rare cancer that few have heard of, unless they or their family have been impacted by the condition. The book provides an overview and explanation of mesothelioma. It also aims to shine a light on the experience of living with mesothelioma, from the perspective of people with it, their families and those who provide support and care.

Chapters outline the challenges of mesothelioma as a rare condition and cover a wide range of issues from diagnosis, treatment, symptom management, psychological impacts, financial implications and the legal process of applying for compensation.

This unique book is informed throughout by the experience-based research conducted by the Mesothelioma UK Research Centre. It is also rooted in the expertise of people from Mesothelioma UK, a charity embedded in the NHS and dedicated to all issues related to the disease. The charity provides a range of information, support and education resources, they fund audit and research and host various events to support the whole mesothelioma community including patients, charities, carers and clinicians.

The charity's flagship service is a team of clinical nurse specialists based strategically across the UK. Each is employed by an NHS hospital but assigned to a cancer alliance with local, regional and national responsibilities. This team of nurses leads and develops specialist mesothelioma services and promotes equitable access to the best treatment and care available for those diagnosed and living with mesothelioma. The nurses have provided, for the first time, a unique, nationwide insight and overview of mesothelioma patient demographics, their experience, and how they are treated and cared for. The close working relationship between the clinical nurse specialists and the research team has informed a dynamic portfolio of patient experience research.

The chapters highlight learning and key messages to emerge from the research cited in the text. The book is practical and accessible to a wide range of readers including people from a health and social care background, people working for charities and the voluntary sector as well as legal professionals working with clients with asbestos-related diseases. It will also be of interest to people with mesothelioma and those close to them. As mesothelioma is a rare disease, the book will have relevance to those working with and affected by other rare conditions.

Acknowledgements

The editors would like to express their thanks to all the contributing authors. We would also like to thank everyone from Mesothelioma UK and the Mesothelioma UK Research Centre at the University of Sheffield who have provided their support. In addition we would like to thank those from other organisations involved in the care and support of people with mesothelioma, who also helped us reach the finishing line. Without this support and encouragement, the book would never have been written.

Most importantly we would like to thank those living with mesothelioma, those with the condition and their families, who shared their experiences and stories. This will enable others to understand the condition and its challenges. We are very grateful for people's generosity in sharing their stories.

Glossary

Actionable tool – an output from a research study which is designed to make a practical improvement, e.g. an information leaflet for patients, a guideline for professionals.

Asbestos Support Group – organisations that provide support and information to people affected by asbestos-related diseases. This includes both the person living with the disease themselves and their informal carers.

BAP-1 – a human gene that produces a protein that helps prevent cancerous tumours grow.

Cancer Alliance – the NHS has established a network of regional Cancer Alliances. Each alliance brings together key organisations in their area to coordinate and improve cancer care locally.

Clinical nurse specialist – a clinical nurse specialist (CNS) is a registered nurse with training and experience in a specific area of nursing. They are often trained to master's level and work at an advanced practice level. In the UK they often have a patient caseload and focus on people with a specific illness or disease such as lung cancer or diabetes.

Coroner – a coroner is a government or judicial officer who investigates deaths, determines the cause of a death and conducts inquests where appropriate. In Scotland the coroner role is conducted by the procurator fiscal.

Co-production – a research approach where the people who will use and benefit from a study collaborate with the researchers to enhance its relevance and usefulness.

Ecotherapy – various types of nature-based methods which increase physical and particularly psychological wellbeing, including self-help activities.

Healthcare professional (HCP) – anyone who has a professional qualification/registration in healthcare, including nurses, doctors, pharmacists, physiotherapists, clinical psychologists.

Indwelling pleural catheter (IPC) – a plastic tube placed under the skin and into the chest cavity that can be left in place for several months so that fluid can be drained on a regular basis.

Inquest – a judicial inquiry conducted to determine the cause of death where this is unknown.

Informal carer – anyone who provides unpaid care for a person requiring support, e.g. spouse, partner, family member, friend or neighbour.

Malignant pleural effusion (MPE) – a condition where fluid builds up in the pleural space around the outside of the lung, beneath the rib cage, causing breathlessness.

Mixed-methods study – a research study combining more than one method for example statistical data and interview data to give a rounded view.

Multidisciplinary team (MDT) – a group of trained staff from different health professions who meet together regularly to discuss the care of individual patients and consider the appropriate care and treatment.

Neuropathic pain – pain that occurs when the nervous system is damaged. The pain can range from mild to severe and is often described as burning, tingling, sharp, stabbing or shooting.

Neutropenia – a condition that occurs when someone has a low level of neutrophils – a type of white blood cell that helps fight infection. Many cancer treatments cause neutropenia.

Neutropenic sepsis – if someone with neutropenia has an infection it is called neutropenic sepsis. This can be life threatening.

Non-expandable lung – also known as "trapped lung", a condition where the lung is unable to expand fully due to tumour encasing its outer lining.

Palliative care – a type of medical care focused on providing relief from the symptoms, pain and stress of a serious illness – whatever the diagnosis may be. Its goal is not to cure the illness but to improve the quality of life for both the patient and their family. It can be provided alongside curative treatments and at any stage of illness, not just at the end of life.

Patient and Public Involvement (PPI) – a process of involving as partners throughout the research process people who have a personal knowledge of and interest in the topic.

Peripheral neuropathy – when the nerves outside of the brain (for example the hands and feet) are damaged or not working properly peripheral neuropathy can develop. Symptoms depend on which nerves are affected.

Pleura – the outer lining of the lung, separated into two layers: visceral (next to the lung) and parietal (underneath the ribs).

Posttraumatic growth (PTG) – positive personal growth resulting from psychological trauma, experienced in one or more of five dimensions: new possibilities, relating to others, personal strength, spiritual change and appreciation of life.

Posttraumatic stress disorder (PTSD) – a mental health condition brought on by experiencing or witnessing a highly frightening or distressing event.

Prognosis – the expected development of a disease, including whether symptoms may get worse and how fast; how quality of life may change; and potential life expectancy.

Psychological intervention – anything which improves mental health and wellbeing for patients and carers, including formal interventions (e.g. medication, psychotherapy) and informal activities, e.g. gardening, singing, talking with friends.

Quality of life (QoL) – a measure of someone's wellbeing. It includes physical, emotional and social wellbeing and acknowledges the impact of wealth, environment and relationships on wellbeing.

Scanxiety – distress and anxiety patients and carers may experience while waiting for a medical imaging scan, during the scan and/or while waiting for results.

Systemic anticancer therapy (SACT) – drugs to treat cancer, including chemotherapy, immunotherapy and targeted therapies.

Talc pleurodesis – the use of medical-grade talc to stick the two layers of pleura together to prevent fluid building up between them (i.e. MPE).

Talc poudrage – medical grade talc sprayed across the pleural surfaces during a surgical thoracoscopy.

Thoracoscopy – a procedure performed under sedation where a camera is inserted into the chest cavity to inspect the pleura, take biopsies and drain fluid.

Traumatic stress symptoms (TSS) – psychological symptoms experienced after a traumatic experience, e.g. flashbacks, nightmares, dissociation, avoidance, irritability, guilt and isolation.

Chapter 1
Introduction

Angela Tod and Clare Gardiner

INTRODUCTION

This book focuses on the experience of living with mesothelioma from the perspective of those with the illness and those close to them. This introductory chapter provides background information about mesothelioma, explains why a book on the experience of living with mesothelioma is required, and why experience-based research is so important. Finally, a brief overview of the book structure and content is provided to help people navigate the text.

This book is intended for a broad audience, although the health and wellbeing needs of the person with mesothelioma is central. In addition to people from a health profession, we aim for it to be relevant to others including social care, the voluntary and charitable sectors, as well as legal professionals, who may all find something interesting to read and learn. In addition, we anticipate that people actually living with mesothelioma and their families may be drawn to the book and find it helpful.

Much of the book is drawn from research conducted in the United Kingdom (UK). For this reason, the UK is our country of focus. However, where appropriate and available, we will draw on international research and information.

MESOTHELIOMA

Mesothelioma is a cancer of the mesothelium, a layer of tissue that surrounds organs such as the pleura and peritoneum. About 80% of cases affect the pleura (the lining of the lung). It is currently incurable. The 5-year survival is 12%, much lower than that for other cancers (Huang et al., 2023). In 2017 there were approximately 34,615 new cases of mesothelioma identified globally, and 29,909

DOI: 10.4324/9781032631318-1

deaths (Zhai et al., 2021). The UK has amongst the highest rates of mesothelioma per capita, a legacy of its asbestos importation and use.

For many years treatments for mesothelioma were limited but more recently new and emerging treatments offer the possibility of living longer with the disease. In the majority of cases mesothelioma is caused by exposure to asbestos. Symptoms and a diagnosis can occur many years after exposure. This can make it difficult for people in terms of understanding the diagnosis and why it occurred. The range and severity of symptoms make a huge impact on people's quality of life and create challenges in terms of treatment and symptom management.

At its heart this book is committed to giving people a voice. It aims to highlight what it is like to have a rare and challenging disease such as mesothelioma. However, issues raised here are transferable to other rare conditions and illnesses with complex symptom clusters.

This book is written by people working in or with the Mesothelioma UK Research Centre (MURC) at the University of Sheffield in England. The MURC is a specialist research centre with expertise in experience-based research. Since July 2020, MURC has been funded by the charity Mesothelioma UK. This charity aims to provide support and information to those with mesothelioma and their families. They have a network of specialist nurses working across the UK and provide a range of resources and services for those affected by mesothelioma. The partnership between the MURC and Mesothelioma UK enables research to be fed immediately into practice and timely change to be made to the way services are provided by the charity and other organisations associated with it, for example specialist legal firms and Asbestos Support Groups.[1]

WHY DO WE NEED A BOOK ON LIVING WITH MESOTHELIOMA?

What is it about mesothelioma that demands such attention and merits a book on the experience of living with it? In addition to its rare nature, the impact of symptoms and the latency period (the gap between asbestos exposure and symptoms), there are other features that create unique challenges for the person with mesothelioma and their families and friends.

Mesothelioma is a rare condition, and many people will not have heard of it prior to diagnosis. Health professionals, such as general physicians and those in primary/community care, may not see anyone with mesothelioma during their career. This creates problems in gaining access to a timely diagnosis and to treatment.

It was previously thought that asbestos-related diseases such as mesothelioma may reduce in number as imports in and the management of asbestos containing products are either banned or better controlled. Importing, supply and use of asbestos was banned in the UK in 1999. Despite this the anticipated decline in the incidence of mesothelioma has not occurred as expected. In addition, there is an indication that who is getting mesothelioma is changing. Prior to the asbestos ban those at risk were involved in the supply or use of asbestos containing materials e.g. dockyard, factory and construction workers. More recently there has been an increase in cases where people have been exposed from the ageing buildings they work or live in (Almark et al., 2023). It is therefore important to understand the experiences and needs of these new populations being diagnosed with mesothelioma.

New treatments for mesothelioma are emerging, it is therefore imperative to gain insight into people's experience of receiving them. In this way the support required for people receiving new treatments, and their families, can be generated and fed back to services. Some recent novel treatments have extended life expectancy for those who respond well, for example immunotherapies. This means more people are living longer with mesothelioma, but we know little about what ongoing care and surveillance is best for long-term survivors, or those participating in clinical trials evaluating new treatments.

As identified above the symptom burden for mesothelioma is high. Common symptoms are breathlessness, pain, cough and fatigue. Whilst these are experienced by people with other conditions, in mesothelioma the symptoms can be hard to treat, and have both a psychological and physical impact (Ejegi-Memeh et al., 2022).

The long time from asbestos exposure to symptoms and diagnosis creates a unique challenge in mesothelioma. When symptoms occur, they may not make sense and may not be linked to the exposure. This can lead to diagnostic delay. In addition, people can struggle to come to terms with the diagnosis as they try and identify where asbestos exposure occurred. For some who work in industries with a legacy of mesothelioma, such as construction and shipbuilding, they may know parents, siblings or work colleagues who have died from the disease. Experiences such as this can mean people live in fear of developing the disease, or fear of the symptoms they witnessed others suffering from.

People with mesothelioma may be eligible for welfare benefits or compensation. In the UK, people diagnosed with mesothelioma can claim Industrial Injuries Disablement Benefit (IIDB) in addition to more generic benefits and allowances such as attendance allowance or personal independence payments. IIDB is paid to people whose illness is caused by asbestos exposure at work. There is also an opportunity to claim compensation through the state or a civil claim. Accessing benefits and compensation can have a positive financial impact for the person with mesothelioma and their family. It can also be seen as a way of highlighting the injustice underlying the illness. However, the process for claiming benefits and/or compensation can be demanding and requires specialist welfare or legal support.

As the above summary demonstrates, there are a myriad of reasons why mesothelioma is an illness with unique challenges that requires the focus and information that a book such as this provides.

EXPERIENCE-BASED RESEARCH

The aim of experience-based research is to capture people's stories and experiences. The research findings are then used in a variety of ways to improve services and inform related policy. Experience-based research is used increasingly in health services and can also be a helpful source of information for people living with a health condition as they strive to understand the impact it will have on their lives and bodies.

Experience-based research tends to employ methods such as surveys, interviews and diaries at one point in time or over a period of time (longitudinally). The Mesothelioma UK Research Centre uses these methods to capture the experiences of people with mesothelioma, and also the experiences of family members and service providers.

Since 2020 the MURC has conducted a portfolio of research studies and developed a reputation of using the study findings to impact on policy and practice. It is this work, and that of our collaborators, that forms the basis for this book.

THE BOOK

The first three chapters of the book will start by providing context regarding mesothelioma. After this introductory chapter, Chapter 2 will explain in more detail what mesothelioma is and why it occurs. The book will then profile the range of experiences across the patient pathway, highlighting the implications of the care delivered by professionals and staff in healthcare, social care and the charitable/voluntary sector. The content will be of relevance for nursing. Mesothelioma UK's team of clinical nurse specialists are world leaders in terms of the organisation of the workforce and their expertise. Research has indicated that the mesothelioma specific clinical nurse specialist (CNS) has a central role in ensuring the care for patients with mesothelioma is accessible, appropriate and timely. Chapter 3 will therefore explain the role of the mesothelioma clinical nurse specialist in the context of multidisciplinary and partnership working.

After these initial chapters the substantial content of the book is presented (Chapters 4 to 10). Here, evidence that relates to the patient experience across the pathway is presented, from diagnosis through to end of life and bereavement. In these chapters a brief description of the topic providing a focus for the chapter is given. This is followed by evidence highlighting the lived experience of the person with mesothelioma and their families. Finally key messages for practice to emerge from the evidence is presented.

The concluding chapters (Chapters 11 to 13) focus on some specific issues where the mesothelioma experience is unique. These are the role of primary care, mental health and wellbeing and the financial and legal aspects of mesothelioma.

CONCLUSION

In this chapter we have provided a brief explanation of mesothelioma as well as experience-based research. We then explained why a book on living with mesothelioma is justified. It concluded with a summary of the book structure and content. Whilst the content of this book is focused on mesothelioma, issues raised here are transferable to other rare and not so rare conditions and illnesses with complex symptom clusters.

NOTE

1   In the UK Asbestos Support Groups are charitable organisations that offer advice and support to people with asbestos-related diseases, including advice on accessing benefits and compensation.

REFERENCES

Almark, P., Tod, A. & Taylor, B. (2023) *The hidden danger of asbestos in UK schools: "I don't think they realise how much risk it poses to students"*. Available at: https://theconversation.com/the-hidden-danger-of-asbestos-in-uk-schools-i-dont-think-they-realise-how-much-risk-it-poses-to-students-203582

Ejegi-Memeh, S., Taylor, B., Tod, A.M., Gardiner, G., Forde, F., Creech, L. & Darlison, L. (2022). Patients' and informal carers' experience of living with mesothelioma: A systematic rapid review and synthesis of the literature. *European Journal of Oncology Nursing*. https://doi.org/10.1016/j.ejon.2022.102122

Huang, J., et al. (2023). Global incidence, risk factors, and temporal trends of mesothelioma: A population-based study. *Journal of Thoracic Oncology*, 18(6), 792–802. https://doi.org/10.1016/j.jtho.2023.01.095

Zhai, Z., et al. (2021). Assessment of global trends in the diagnosis of mesothelioma from 1990 to 2017. *JAMA Network Open*, 4(8), p. e2120360. https://doi.org/10.1001/jamanetworkopen.2021.20360

Chapter 2

Mesothelioma

Leah Taylor, Peter Allmark and Angela Tod

OVERVIEW

Mesothelioma is a public health disaster. The United Kingdom (UK) has the highest incidence of the disease globally which is reflective of the manufacture and use of asbestos products over decades. This chapter will briefly discuss the global perspective of asbestos then focus on the UK use of asbestos and link to mesothelioma. Three waves of mesothelioma will be described: 1) early years: workers in mining, manufacture and movement of asbestos; 2) post-WW2 high-risk occupations e.g. construction/shipbuilding; and 3) exposure from buildings containing asbestos.

Mesothelioma risk has long been associated with heavy industry with the belief that the disease mainly affected older men who had worked in high-risk occupations. Here, these perceptions are challenged, drawing upon data from national audits and research into groups thought to be less at risk such as healthcare workers and education workers. The chapter will explore the incidence and experience of mesothelioma and asbestos exposure among different groups, for example, veterans, healthcare, education, highlighting the common and unique experiences. The gendered implications of occupational risk will also be considered.

The pathology of mesothelioma will be described, how the disease develops and the different subtypes, whilst pleural mesothelioma is most common, peritoneal, testicular and pericardial mesothelioma will also be addressed.

The implications of living with a mesothelioma diagnosis are discussed, raising some of the complexities and challenges patients and families face. This will preface the chapters to follow which discuss, in depth, issues of symptom burden, disease impact, lack of treatment options, access to clinical trials, legal and financial issues and equitable access to treatment and care.

DOI: 10.4324/9781032631318-2

The chapter will conclude by drawing on existing evidence to provide recommendations for practice to raise awareness of mesothelioma and how understanding the lived experience of patients with mesothelioma is important to meet care and support needs.

THE EVIDENCE

The history of asbestos use and disease/mesothelioma

The link between asbestos and mesothelioma is exceptionally strong. There are few other known causes, and these are rare and geographically specific, for example, to southeast Turkey (Demirer, 2015). Outside these areas, asbestos is almost certainly the cause, even if the exposure is unknown.

In the UK, commercial asbestos use began in the 1870s as protection against high temperatures in steam-powered industries. It was later used as a fire retardant and heat insulator in buildings. The first recorded deaths due to asbestos were of lung fibrosis, in 1899 and 1924. Regulations to control exposure were introduced in 1931 (Taylor, 2018). The use of asbestos, however, continued unabated. The period of maximum importation and use of asbestos in Western Europe was 1920–1970; and the UK was the highest importer within that group (Kameda et al., 2014). This was mainly due to its ability to import cheaply from colonies and former colonies (Pickles, 2018).

By 1960 it was clear that asbestos was linked to lung cancer and, notably, to the previously almost unknown cancer, mesothelioma (Anon, 2000). Furthermore, patients were not all heavily exposed to asbestos; just living near an asbestos factory or living with someone who worked with asbestos caused sufficient exposure.

The road to an eventual ban on the use of asbestos in UK construction was long; its ban in 1999 came after bans in France and Germany but predated the EU-wide ban of 2005. Many countries still permit mining or use of asbestos, including China and the United States. Pre-1999 buildings in the UK may contain asbestos; for example, it is estimated that over 80% of UK schools have asbestos "present on their estate" (DfE, 2019).

Changing face of mesothelioma

Following the 1999 ban, it was expected that rates of mesothelioma would gradually decline in the UK. There are indications that this process has begun

(HSE, 2023). One issue, however, is whether the legacy of asbestos in UK buildings, especially as they deteriorate, poses a risk to those working in or regularly using them.

In the main, the official statistics (e.g. HSE/ONS data) on deaths by occupation have yet to pick up any such trend. Peto et al. found increased risk of mesothelioma only in heavy industries that used asbestos, such as construction, but none in occupations where people worked in buildings containing asbestos, such as teaching or nursing (Peto et al., 2009). There are several concerns with this official data (Taylor et al., 2023; 2024).

- The data records only the final occupation; those who move from teaching to, say, care work will not be recorded as former teachers.
- Deaths over age 75 are not recorded by former occupation. Mesothelioma has a long latency from exposure to asbestos. Many deaths in this older group will nonetheless be the result of exposure at work.
- Many workers are not included in the data. A review (Taylor et al., 2022) looking at media reports of former school workers with mesothelioma found that 19 of the 84 cases were non-teaching staff, including caretakers, cleaners and dinner ladies. These would not be shown in the data used by Peto et al. (2009) and others.
- Many are not included in the data, most importantly, pupils in schools who could be exposed throughout their school life. It is known that the lifetime risk is highest in those whose exposure occurs when young (Committee on Carcinogenicity of Chemicals in Food Consumer Products and the Environment, 2013). Modelling in the USA suggests that nine pupils will develop mesothelioma for each education worker who does so (Environmental Protection Agency (USA), 1980). Recent work suggests the risk to pupils is even greater (JUAC, 2021).
- There has been a more-than doubling in UK mesothelioma deaths amongst the under 40s: 2008–17 there were 2.7 deaths per annum; 2017–21 there were 6.26 per annum (HSE/ONS, n.d.); although these numbers are small it is likely to be an indicator of increasing risk to pupils (Marinaccio, 2015).
- Freedom of Information requests have shown that the rates of mesothelioma measured, for example, by those taking industrial injury benefits, are several times higher than the official data suggests (Taylor et al., 2023; 2024). Taking the official death statistics as they stand, in 2023 it was noteworthy that education professionals now lead the table of occupational groups for mesothelioma deaths in females.

These concerns lend weight to the belief that the UK is facing a third wave of mesothelioma. The first wave affected those mining and manufacturing asbestos, the second, those working with it directly or those nearby, and the third, those using buildings containing asbestos that is insufficiently contained (Emmett and Cakouos, 2017).

Those working with mesothelioma patients, including charities and specialist health workers, say that previously people with mesothelioma were overwhelmingly male and working in heavy industry or construction. Now they see an increasing proportion of women who have often worked in areas such as education and healthcare. Recent research has examined the experiences of healthcare workers (Mesothelioma Asbestos Guidance Study, MAGS) (Allmark et al., 2020), education workers (Mesothelioma Education Workers Study, MEWS) (Taylor et al., 2022) and of women (Gendered Experience of Mesothelioma Study, GEMS) (Ejegi-Memeh et al., 2021). One key finding of these studies is that the experiences of such groups are different from those working where asbestos exposure risk is high. For example, diagnosis can be slower as clinicians have a low index of suspicion of mesothelioma in such patients. The research also showed that large numbers of former hospital and school workers who developed mesothelioma were not counted in the official data used to estimate asbestos risk. As such, the risk to school and hospital workers is greatly underestimated.

Mesothelioma as a disease

Mesothelioma is a rare disease. It accounts for less than 1% of cancer cases in the UK (CRUK, n.d.). However, mesothelioma is a devastating diagnosis presenting unique challenges for those diagnosed, their loved ones and the healthcare community.

Mesothelioma is a cancer which forms in the membranes (mesothelium) that line the chest and abdomen covering some of the internal organs in both cavities. Within the chest the mesothelium is called the pleura and within the abdomen is it called the peritoneum. When this cancer occurs, it is referred to as pleural and peritoneal mesothelioma respectively.

Pleural mesothelioma accounts for almost 90% of all cases, peritoneal mesothelioma for approximately 10%. The disease can isolate itself to the pericardium and testicles, this latter form of mesothelioma accounts for less than 1%. Overall, more men are affected by mesothelioma, however, more women develop peritoneal disease than pleural. In the UK the median age of patients diagnosed with pleural and peritoneal mesothelioma is 76 years and 71 years respectively. Whilst mesothelioma is reported to be rare in younger populations it does occur in people under 70 years of age

Pleural mesothelioma

The pleura is a two-layered membrane, the outer layer lining the chest wall is called the parietal pleura and the inner layer the visceral pleura (see Figure 2.1). These are serous membranes which produce a small amount of fluid reducing friction between lungs and pleura during the movement of breathing. Mesothelioma develops on the parietal pleura first, growing nodules which eventually combine to form a larger tumour. As the disease progresses it will extend to involve the visceral pleura (Brims, 2021). Mesothelioma can cause fluid to build up between the two pleural linings, known as a pleural effusion.

Pleural mesothelioma typically presents with the patient experiencing progressive breathlessness. In addition, there may be fatigue, weight loss and pain, particularly localised to the affected chest wall. The breathlessness in mesothelioma results from pleural effusion (fluid building up between the lung and its lining) and/or thickened pleura restricting expansion of the lung during breathing.

In the UK most pleural and some peritoneal mesothelioma is managed by specialist lung cancer teams, however, mesothelioma is not lung cancer. It has its own distinct morphology, pattern of growth, response and resistance to treatment.

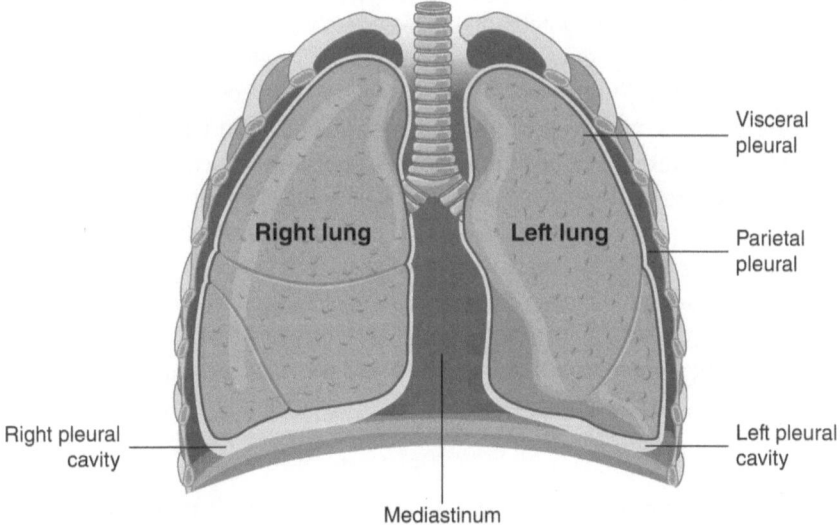

Figure 2.1 Pleural mesothelioma

At the beginning of the diagnostic process most patients will have a chest x-ray which may show presence of pleural thickening or a pleural effusion, however, in early stages of the disease these can be undetectable (see Chapter 4). Where there is suspicion of malignancy a detailed scan will be undertaken using computerised tomography (CT), often referred to as a CT scan. A CT scan provides cross-sectional images of the chest enabling the radiologist to determine if pleural thickening and or pleural effusion is present and extent of disease. magnetic resonance imaging (MRI) and positron emission tomography (PET) are occasionally used in diagnosis, but their role is less well established in routine practice.

A tissue biopsy is of utmost importance in distinguishing mesothelioma from other types of cancer. A biopsy can be obtained by either a core biopsy under the guidance of a CT or ultrasound scan, more invasive methods include thoracoscopy under general anaesthetic or sedation. Tests used depend upon availability, extent of disease and health of the patient. In the laboratory immunohistochemistry tests are performed on biopsy specimens to determine malignancy and establish the subtype of mesothelioma.

Mesothelioma has three distinct subtypes, epithelioid, sarcomatoid and biphasic (a mix of the two previous subtypes). Determining subtype will indicate likely progression of the disease and potential for response to treatment (see Chapter 5). Epithelioid disease usually has a better response to chemotherapy and a more favourable prognosis. Sarcomatoid disease often behaves more aggressively. It can respond well to immunotherapy, but less so to chemotherapy. In biphasic disease, the weighting between the two subtypes will determine whether the disease is more likely to behave like the epithelioid or sarcomatoid subtype. Mesothelioma is a heterogeneous tumour meaning that all areas are unlikely to be the same. Taking biopsies from one area of disease may not give the full diagnostic picture, for example, epithelioid disease may be found on biopsy from one area but it is possible there are areas of biphasic disease elsewhere. Where possible it is preferable for the patient to undergo thoracoscopy so that larger samples of tissue can be taken. Clinicians are beginning to understand that exploration of mesothelioma at a molecular level can give additional information to guide healthcare teams and patients and help with discussions about prognosis. This is a new and emerging field that will continue to develop in the future.

Mesothelioma is a progressive disease. The pleura continues to thicken as the disease grows within causing a likely increase in symptoms such as breathlessness, pain, weight loss and fatigue due to bulk of tumour and systemic burden of disease (see Chapter 6). Mesothelioma is sometimes thought to be localised within the pleura, however, studies have shown high rates of both intra and extra thoracic metastases (Finn et al., 2012). It is important that healthcare teams are aware of this when caring for patients.

Pleural mesothelioma is staged using the International Association for the Study of Lung Cancer (IASLC) TNM classification of mesothelioma. This staging system determines extent of disease using the tumour, nodes, metastases descriptors which can guide prognosis. Currently staging for mesothelioma is different from other cancers, where different stages will determine treatment regimens suitable for that stage of disease. In mesothelioma the recommended treatment is the same regardless of stage. Recording staging and identifying early disease remains important, especially in the context of clinical trials, particularly where more radical treatments are being used. In the UK staging is required as part of the national dataset and was a recommendation of the British Thoracic Society (BTS) guideline for the investigation and management of pleural mesothelioma (BTS, 2018). Despite this, data completeness remains an issue with the National Mesothelioma Audit 2020 reporting only 65% of patients had disease stage recorded (Royal College of Physicians (RCP), 2020b).

Peritoneal mesothelioma

The peritoneum is a two-layered membrane which lines the abdominal cavity. Its function is to protect and support abdominal organs, conducting the passage of blood vessels and nerves. The outer layer which is attached to the abdominal wall is called the parietal peritoneum. The inner layer, called the visceral peritoneum, wraps around internal organs such as the stomach, spleen and parts of the bowel. The peritoneum produces fluid to lubricate and reduce friction allowing the abdominal organs to move against each other. The peritoneum is formed of mesothelial cells (see Figure 2.2).

Mesothelioma causes the peritoneum to thicken which can often be seen using a CT scan Asking patients to drink a contrast prior to their CT scan is recommend as this helps image the peritoneum and its proximity to the small bowel more accurately. This can determine feasibility of surgical options. CT scanning will also guide healthcare teams about possible sites to obtain a biopsy to confirm diagnosis. This is of critical importance in distinguishing mesothelioma from other types of cancer. Overaccumulation of fluid in the abdomen is called ascites. Sampling this fluid has been shown to be of limited benefit.

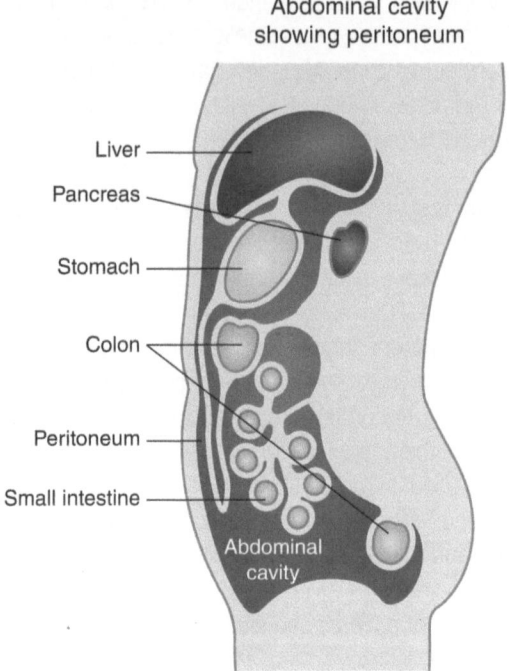

Figure 2.2 Peritoneal mesothelioma

The term peritoneal mesothelioma represents a spectrum of subtypes. At the lower end of the spectrum there is multicystic mesothelioma and well-differentiated papillary mesothelial tumours. At the other end the more aggressive diffuse malignant peritoneal mesothelioma subtypes are epithelioid, sarcomatoid and biphasic. Most cases diagnosed are epithelioid.

There is no official staging system for peritoneal mesothelioma. Peritoneal doctors and radiologists use the peritoneal cancer index (PCI) system. Using the index the abdomen is divided into 13 regions and given a score if tumour is found in that region. The PCI is calculated by adding together the regions. The maximum score is 39, with a higher PCI suggesting wider spread of disease.

People with peritoneal mesothelioma can present with vague symptoms such as distention, abdominal pain, altered bowel habit, anorexia, weight loss and fatigue. Sometimes symptoms will precede diagnosis by months or even years. The vague nature of symptoms and the rarity of peritoneal mesothelioma can lead to a delay in the diagnosis being made. Abdominal pain and distension are the most frequently reported symptoms. As the disease progresses towards end of life, the patient may experience uncontrolled ascites or intestinal obstruction.

Challenges of living with mesothelioma

Living with mesothelioma can present some unique and complex challenges for the patient and those close to them. A systematic review reported high levels of both physical and psychological burden (Ejegi-Memeh et al., 2022). Many of the issues facing patients and families directly, such as psychological wellbeing, symptom management, legal and financial implications of a diagnosis and involvement of the coroner in deaths will be discussed in detail throughout the book. The remainder of this chapter will discuss some wider organisational and service limitations which can cause additional challenge and burden for patients, families and healthcare teams.

The rarity of mesothelioma can itself present some unique challenges. Patients with rare cancers may suffer worse quality of life and higher levels of loneliness and anxiety (Duijts and van der Zwan, 2021) and those diagnosed with poor prognosis cancers report poorer experiences of care (Alessy et al., 2022). Whilst there are regions with a high incidence of mesothelioma linked to past industry, patients with mesothelioma are generally spread throughout the UK. Those living in areas with a high incidence of the disease are more likely to have access to specialist knowledge and expertise whilst those in areas with fewer diagnoses may have a greater challenge in this regard. Standards of care and possibly outcomes have close correlation with the organisation of services and the resources available (RCP, 2020b).

Variation in mesothelioma care and treatment may be underpinned by experience and knowledge (Henshall et al., 2022). Clinicians who had little experience of treating patients with mesothelioma were likely to be more nihilistic in their attitude due to the lack of treatment options and perceived lack of usefulness. Lack of specialist care and variation in treatment present challenges for patients and families who look to their healthcare teams to provide them with the best advice for treatment based upon the latest evidence.

In 2013 the Mesothelioma Service Specifications were published for England (NHS England, 2103), outlining the need for regional specialist mesothelioma multidisciplinary teams (MDT) to provide specialised advice. It was envisaged teams would be formed of MDT members, often from a lung cancer MDT, with a specialist interest and expertise in the disease. The remit of the mesothelioma MDT included providing expert care for diagnosis and management, access to an experienced clinical nurse specialist and ensuring local/regional protocols were in place to make certain all patients had access to relevant clinical trials.

In 2019 the National Mesothelioma Audit identified 15 specialist MDTs operating across England. It highlighted variation in referral, information offered and access to support. However, patients referred to those specialist MDTs were found to be more likely to benefit from access to a dedicated mesothelioma clinical nurse specialist and have increased access to clinical trials within their local area (RCP, 2020a). Whilst the report clearly shows some progress in this area, the MDTs were self-identified and based in individual hospitals, rather than being the established regionwide service that was commissioned by the NHS. Furthermore, several regions in England have no access to a specialist MDT at all. Scotland has a nationally funded mesothelioma network and MDT.

A potential benefit of specialist teams and MDTs is that they provide opportunities to continuously upskill and increase knowledge of other healthcare professionals about new and upcoming developments in treatment and trials. This aims to improve access to specialist mesothelioma clinical decision-making, treatment and trials.

Within the UK several patient networks exist on social media. On these platforms patients and carers often ask questions of their peers regarding mesothelioma specialists. They are prepared to self-refer, travelling hundreds of miles from their home to access specialist care in the hope of more options than those available to them locally.

As highlighted above, there remains a persistence in the belief that mesothelioma is associated with male-dominated heavy industry. This contributes to a low index of suspicion for some. Hence a GP might be less likely to suspect mesothelioma in a woman than a man, and in a teacher than a builder. Those involved in the care of patients with mesothelioma, and those involved in health and safety work need to adapt to this change. Initiatives such as the Scottish Mesothelioma Network are one example of how this can happen.

IMPLICATIONS FOR POLICY/PRACTICE

In the UK there is an increasing body of evidence detailing the lived experience of people with and affected by mesothelioma in addition to nationally collected data on incidence, treatment and survival.

Increasing awareness of mesothelioma among health professionals is a continued challenge. Due to its rarity many general practitioners will see very few or no mesothelioma cases in their practice. This can pose a barrier to early detection and recognition of the unique needs of this patient group. The continued use of asbestos globally in addition to the amount of asbestos which persists in buildings throughout the UK affirms this disease will be present for generations to come. Asbestos-related diseases, including mesothelioma, should be included in the curriculum for undergraduate doctors and nurses to lower their index of suspicion and ensure it is not thought of as a disease of the past. There is no accredited education programme available for mesothelioma, at best mesothelioma forms part of the curriculum of courses on lung cancer and respiratory medicine. Developing accessible accredited education resources would ensure those caring for patients could significantly enhance their knowledge.

Charities operate at local and national levels, advocating for improvements and ensuring the patient voice is central to development of services. However, their impact can be limited by the availability of resources and their ability to influence wider policy. Much of the work undertaken to understand the lived experience of mesothelioma has been funded by charities such as Mesothelioma UK. To make real change policymakers and commissioners must ensure they work in collaboration with such organisations to ensure services meet the needs of those who so critically need them.

Studies mentioned earlier such as MAGS, MEWS and GEMS developed recommendations from their findings. Some of these recommendations have been cited above. At the diagnostic level, clinicians should be aware of the potential for mesothelioma in women and in those working in non-traditional industries, as well as those in high-risk occupations. Regarding awareness and education, staff working in areas such as schools and hospitals containing asbestos need to have asbestos awareness included in their mandatory training and health and safety modules. At government level, there is discussion over whether the UK policy on asbestos in the public estate should continue to be that of management in situ. There is a proposal that a deadline should be set for its removal. Many EU countries have far stricter policies on monitoring and removal of asbestos. There are also moves towards a phased removal of asbestos from public buildings in the EU (European Commission, 2022). Government policy is based on ONS data which the research cited here suggests is a gross underestimate of actual levels of mesothelioma in those working in areas such as hospitals and schools. For this reason, charities such as Mesothelioma UK and the education and healthcare unions generally favour the phased removal policy.

CONCLUSION

This chapter has introduced mesothelioma. It has explained the causes and changing nature of the population developing the disease. It has also provided an overview of the disease, how it develops in the body and some of the challenges for people with the disease. Many of the issues raised will be discussed in more detail in the following chapters of the book.

REFERENCES

Alessy, S., et al. (2022). Factors influencing cancer patients' experiences of care in the USA, United Kingdom, and Canada: A systematic review. *eClinicalMedicine*, 47. Available at: https://www.thelancet.com/journals/eclinm/article/PIIS2589-5370(22)00135-3/fulltext (Accessed 16 September 2024)

Allmark, P., Tod, A.M. & Darlison, L. (2020). *MAGS: The Healthcare Staff Mesothelioma Asbestos Guidance Study*. Available at: https://www.mesothelioma.uk.com/past-research-projects/#mags (Accessed: 16 August 2024)

Anon (2000). Obituary: Christopher Wagner. *The Telegraph*, 12 July. Available at: https://www.telegraph.co.uk/news/health/1347992/Christopher-Wagner.html (Accessed: 16 August 2024)

Brims, F. (2021). Epidemiology and clinical aspects of malignant pleural mesothelioma. *Cancers (Basel)*, 13(16), p. 4194.

BTS (2018). *BTS guideline for the investigation and management of pleural mesothelioma*. Available at: https://www.brit-thoracic.org.uk/quality-improvement/guidelines/mesothelioma/ (Accessed 16 September 2024)

Cancer Research UK (CRUK) (n.d.). *Mesothelioma incidence statistics*. Available at: https://www.cancerresearchuk.org/health-professional/cancer-statistics/statistics-by-cancer-type/mesothelioma/incidence (Accessed: 16 August 2024)

Committee on Carcinogenicity of Chemicals in Food Consumer Products and the Environment (2013). *Relative vulnerability of children to asbestos compared to adults*. Available at: https://www.gov.uk/government/publications/relative-vulnerability-of-children-to-asbestos-compared-to-adults

Demirer, E., et al. (2015). Clinical and prognostic features of erionite-induced malignant mesothelioma. *Yonsei Medical Journal*, 56(2), pp. 311–323.

Department for Education (DfE) (2019). *Asbestos Management Assurance Process (AMAP) report*. Available at: https://assets.publishing.service.gov.uk/government/uploads/system/uploads/attachment_data/file/906343/AMAP_Report_2019.pdf (Accessed: 16 August 2024)

Duijts, F. & Maarten van der Zwan, J. (2021). Rare cancer and cancer of unknown primary: Here's what you should know! *European Journal of Cancer Care*, 30. https://doi.org/10.1111/ecc.13508

Ejegi-Memeh S., et al. (2021). Gender and the experiences of living with mesothelioma. *European Journal of Oncology Nursing*, 52. https://doi.org/10.1016/j.ejon.2021.101966

Ejegi-Memeh, S., et al. (2022). Patients' and informal carers' experience of living with mesothelioma: A systematic rapid review and synthese of the literature. *European Journal of Oncology Nursing*, 58. https://doi.org/10.1016/j.ejon.2022.102122

Emmett, E. & Cakouros, B. (2017). Communities at high risk in the third wave of mesothelioma. In J. Testa (ed.), *Asbestos and mesothelioma*. London: Springer International, pp.103–130.

Environmental Protection Agency (USA) (1980). *Support document for proposed rule on friable asbestos-containing materials in schools: report no. 560/12-80-003*. Available at: https://nepis.epa.gov/Exe/ZyNET.exe/9100BENP.TXT?ZyActionD=ZyDocument&Client=EPA&

Index=1976+Thru+1980&Docs=&Query=&Time=&EndTime=&SearchMethod=1&TocRestrict
=n&Toc=&TocEntry=&QField=&QFieldYear=&QFieldMonth=&QFieldDay=&IntQFieldOp=0&E
xtQFieldOp=0&XmlQuery=&File=D%3A%5Czyfiles%5CIndex%20Data%5C76thru80%5CTxt%
5C00000012%5C9100BENP.txt&User=ANONYMOUS&Password=anonymous&SortMethod=h
%7C-&MaximumDocuments=1&FuzzyDegree=0&ImageQuality=r75g8/r75g8/x150y150g16/
i425&Display=hpfr&DefSeekPage=x&SearchBack=ZyActionL&Back=ZyActionS&BackDes
c=Results%20page&MaximumPages=1&ZyEntry=1&SeekPage=x&ZyPURL (Accessed: 16
August 2024)

European Commission (2022). *Questions and answers: Towards an asbestos-free future*.
Available at: https://ec.europa.eu/commission/presscorner/detail/en/qanda_22_5678
(Accessed: 22 October 2024)

Finn, R.S., Brims, F.J.H., Gandhi, A., Olsen, N., Musk, A.W., Maskell, N.A., & Lee, Y.C.G. (2012).
Postmortem findings of malignant pleural mesothelioma: A two-center study of 318
patients. *Chest*, 142(5), pp. 1267–1273. https://doi.org/10.1378/chest.11-3204

Henshall, C., et al. (2022). Understanding clinical decision-making in mesothelioma care: a
mixed methods study. *BMJ Open Respiratory Research*, 9(1). https://doi.org/10.1136%2Fbm
jresp-2022-001312

HSE/Office for National Statistics (n.d.). *Deaths from asbestos-related and other occupational
lung diseases*. Available at: https://www.hse.gov.uk/statistics/tables/index.htm#lung
(Accessed: 16 August 2024)

HSE/Office for National Statistics (2023). *Mesothelioma statistics for Great Britain, 2023*.
Available at: https://www.coniac.org.uk/uploads/mesothelioma.pdf?v=1690278499
(Accessed: 16 August 2024)

Joint Union Asbestos Committee (JUAC) (2021). *Continuing government failure leads to
rise in school mesothelioma deaths*. Available at: https://norac.org.uk/wp-content/
uploads/2021/07/Continuing-Government-Failure-leads-to-rise-in-school-mesothelioma-
deaths-JUAC-REPORT-02-07-2021-FINAL.pdf (Accessed: 16 August 2024)

Kameda, T., et al. (2014). Asbestos: Use, bans and disease burden in Europe. *Bull World Health
Organ*, 92(11), pp. 790–797.

Marinaccio, A., et al. (2015). Malignant mesothelioma due to non-occupational asbestos
exposure from the Italian national surveillance system (ReNaM): Epidemiology and public
health issues. *Occupational and Environmental Medicine*, 72(9), pp. 648–655.

NHS England (2013). *2013/14 NHS standard contract for cancer: Malignant mesothelioma
(adult)*. Available at: https://www.england.nhs.uk/wp-content/uploads/2013/06/b10-cancer-
mal-mesot.pdf (Accessed 16 September 2024)

Peto, J., Rake, C., Gilham, C. & Hatch, J. (2009). *Occupational, domestic and environmental
mesothelioma risks in Britain: A case-control study. RR696*. Health and Safety Executive.

Pickles, C. (2018). *Why the UK needs tighter asbestos controls*. Lucion Services.

RCP (2020a). *National Mesothelioma Audit organisational report 2019*. Available at: https://
mesothelioma.uk.com/wp-content/uploads/dlm_uploads/2021/02/200121_NMA_Meso_
org_report_Final_23Jan20_WEB-002_0_0.pdf (Accessed 16 September 2024)

RCP (2020b). *National Mesothelioma Audit report 2020 (for the audit period 2016–18)*.
Available at: https://www.mesothelioma.uk.com/downloads/national-mesothelioma-audit-
2020/?wpdmdl=15399 (Accessed 16 September 2024)

Taylor, A.N. (2018). The asbestos story: A tale of public health and politics. *Imperial Medicine Blog*, 2 February. Available at: https://blogs.imperial.ac.uk/imperial-medicine/2018/02/02/the-asbestos-story-a-tale-of-public-health-and-politics/ (Accessed: 16 August 2024)

Taylor, B., Allmark, P. & Tod, A. (2022). The experiences of presentation, diagnosis, treatment and care for school-based education workers with mesothelioma: A scoping review. *International Journal of Nursing and Health Care Research*, 5, p.1342. https://doi.org/10.29011/2688-9501.101342

Taylor, B., Allmark, P. & Tod, A. (2023). The hidden danger of asbestos in UK schools: "I don't think they realise how much risk it poses to students". *The Conversation*, 18 April. Available at: https://theconversation.com/the-hidden-danger-of-asbestos-in-uk-schools-i-dont-think-they-realise-how-much-risk-it-poses-to-students-203582 (Accessed: 16 August 2024)

Taylor, B., Allmark, P. & Tod, A. (2024). Mesothelioma caused by asbestos in UK public buildings: An ongoing risk to public health. *People, Place and Policy*. https://doi.org/10.3351/ppp.2024.7668957929

Chapter 3

The role of the specialist nurse in multidisciplinary and partnership working

Leah Taylor, Sarah Hargreaves and Angela Tod

OVERVIEW

This chapter provides an example of how clinical specialist nursing can promote multidisciplinary working and achieve better patient outcomes and experiences in mesothelioma. The example used is the Mesothelioma UK clinical nurse specialist (CNS) nursing team. The mesothelioma community comprises a range of professionals and organisations including charities, academics, support groups, benefits advisors and specialist personal injury lawyers. This chapter will discuss the pivotal partnership role the mesothelioma CNS (MCNS) has in working with these stakeholders to ensure people with mesothelioma receive the very best specialist support and advice.

Threats to the provision and sustainability of the MCNS workforce will be discussed. Challenges such as a lack of central funding, the impact of Covid-19 and recent global financial instability will be addressed. These concerns have limited growth of specialist nursing roles such as the MCNS and impacted on those already in post.

The chapter will conclude with recommendations to mitigate some of the threats to the MCNS role, such as national recognition of the value of the CNS with central financial support to ensure sustainability of the service. A standardised career development framework to promote retention of the workforce and protect the role from being used to plug staffing gaps is also needed. Further research into the value of the CNS role within rare cancers is also needed, building on research evidence conducted by the Mesothelioma Research Centre.

DOI: 10.4324/9781032631318-3

THE EVIDENCE

The development of the CNS role within cancer care

CNS roles were initially introduced in the USA in the 1930s and have developed steadily in the UK since the 1970s in response to gaps in patient care, medical workforce shortages and national policy developments (Castledine, 2002; Barton et al., 2012; Cannaby et al., 2020).

The first CNS roles in the UK were driven through local innovations, developed by nurses. In the 1990s a new generation of CNSs was born out of a need to cover medical staffing pressures, with CNSs taking on a range of roles traditionally associated with medicine (Castledine, 2002). Initially CNS roles were not well defined, with wide variations in educational preparation, role, titles and pay, dependent on the needs of local services. However, there are now consistencies in the role, with most CNSs acting as key workers, contributing to multiprofessional meetings, service development and enhancing patient experience (Cannaby et al., 2020; Leary et al., 2017; Kerr et al., 2021).

In recent years there has been growing evidence of the value of CNS roles in cancer care. Advancing cancer treatments mean people are living longer with and beyond cancer, resulting in complex cancer pathways and a greater spectrum of lasting effects from treatment. Nurses make up the largest part of the cancer workforce and are an integral part of the pathway as they lead and manage patients through diagnosis, treatment, surveillance, supportive and end of life care. The contribution made specifically by CNSs has been difficult to quantify but there is emerging evidence of the value of the role within the pathway (Kerr et al., 2021). Benefits of the CNS role include reducing and avoiding emergency admissions and increased uptake of cancer treatments. Despite financial pressures in healthcare, CNS posts are increasing, although many are fully or partially funded by charities (Macmillan Cancer Support, 2017).

Recent guidance from Health Education England (HEE, 2023) has provided further support and clarity through the Aspirant Cancer Career and Education Development (ACCEND) framework. This sets out a career development pathway for cancer CNSs, incorporating the four pillars of: clinical practice, research, leadership and education. The framework differentiates between those working at an "enhanced level", managing discrete aspects of patient care, and those at an "advanced level", managing whole episodes of care from start to finish (HEE, 2023). Those working at an advanced level can be generalists or specialists and have developed a breadth of knowledge and skills at master's degree level.

With the development of cancer diagnostic and treatment pathways, the role of the CNS has been firmly established as a core member of the multidisciplinary team (MDT) in more common cancers (NHS England, 2024). The first cancer CNS posts were developed in breast cancer care with other tumour groups following suit. Lung cancer CNSs were introduced in the early 2000s, however, unfortunately this did not include investment in specialist mesothelioma CNSs, therefore care traditionally formed part of a lung cancer CNS role (Macmillan Cancer Support, 2017).

Development of the CNS role within mesothelioma

Mesothelioma UK is a charity that supports people with mesothelioma and their families. Mesothelioma UK was established in 2004, with funding from Macmillan Cancer Support (MCS). Initially called the National MCS Mesothelioma Resource Centre (NMMRC) it was based at the University Hospitals of Leicester. NMMRC grew rapidly and became an independent charity in 2008, renamed Mesothelioma UK. The organisation was the vision of Liz Darlison and colleagues, based at the University Hospitals of Leicester. Liz is a Mesothelioma Nurse Consultant, widely regarded as the first specialist mesothelioma nurse in the UK and a pioneer for specialist nursing in rare cancers.

The mission of Mesothelioma UK was to provide equitable access to the best treatment and care possible through the provision of specialist mesothelioma nursing at the point of need. This remains at the heart of the charity's activity today. To achieve this goal, over the past 20 years Mesothelioma UK has funded CNS posts in NHS hospitals ensuring nurses are embedded at the forefront of patient care. Today there are approximately 30 dedicated mesothelioma CNSs funded by the charity through public fundraising, donations from charitable partners and grants (Mesothelioma UK, 2024). This MCNS network is a unique initiative globally. These MCNSs have previous experience in lung cancer, oncology, palliative care and research. Working at the frontline within lung cancer and thoracic oncology multidisciplinary teams, the mesothelioma CNS aims to improve access to the best care and treatment available, including the provision of generalist and some specialist palliative care. The MCNSs form a specialist nursing network reaching across all four nations of the UK.

As nurses working in a rare cancer the scope of the role extends beyond traditional clinical duties, they also act as leaders in the field of mesothelioma nursing. In addition to their patient caseload MCNSs educate and advocate for improvements in care and treatment regionally, nationally and internationally. An example is a highly specialised MCNS who is solely dedicated to the care of patients with peritoneal mesothelioma who works across the breadth of the UK to provide support and improve outcomes for patients.

Mesothelioma UK provides funding to trusts and health boards to host dedicated mesothelioma nursing posts. The nurses are mostly members of lung cancer or pleural teams and are funded to care for patients with mesothelioma for approximately two days a week. The remaining funding for their post is met by the host NHS trust where the nurse continues to meet non-mesothelioma clinical responsibilities. The posts are framed by a service level agreement between Mesothelioma UK and the host NHS trust which sets out the core roles and responsibilities. However, unlike traditional cancer CNS roles the MCNS works at a local, regional and national level. The MCNSs level of practice varies according to the service level agreement with the host organisation, but all work at an enhanced or advanced level of practice (HEE, 2023).

The ambition of Mesothelioma UK is to ensure MCNS posts cover all areas of the UK. Whilst most of the nurses are currently based in England some of the highest rates of mesothelioma occur in Glasgow. Following a successful pilot project between Mesothelioma UK and Macmillan, a team of five MCNSs are now commissioned by NHS Scotland. The Scottish MCNS work strategically as core members of the Scottish Mesothelioma Network and provide geographical cover for Scotland. Wales is a mainly rural country with high levels of deprivation and the incidence of mesothelioma is approximately half that of Scotland (Cancer Research UK, 2024). To date no commissioned MCNS services exist despite a commitment to establish them by NHS Wales. There is currently one funded MCNS for Wales. Northern Ireland has approximately 50 mesothelioma diagnoses per year. To meet that need, the first MCNS role in Northern Ireland will be established in 2024. See Table 3.1 for the average numbers of new cases of mesothelioma per year and number of CNSs in each of the UK countries.

Table 3.1 Number of new cases of mesothelioma per year, per 100,000, in the UK (2017–2019) and number of MCNSs

	Female	Male	Total number of cases	Number of MCNSs
England	410	1939	2349	21
Scotland	27	172	199	4
Wales	17	89	107	1
Northern Ireland	9	44	53	[1 starting in 2024]

(Cancer Research UK, 2024; Mesothelioma UK, 2024)

The remit and role of the MCNS

A strength of the Mesothelioma UK MCNS network is that it works within the NHS, a unified healthcare system free at the point of delivery. Whilst the four nations of the UK NHS systems all operate under their own statutory bodies, the organisation and delivery of services is consistent. Currently in the UK, cancer services are driven by national policy through the NHS Cancer Programme. They are organised at regional level by Cancer Alliances and Networks, monitoring and reporting is undertaken by the National Cancer Registration and Analysis Service (NCRAS) (Public Health England, 2020). This national direction and governance ensure all involved in cancer service delivery are working towards the same goals. Within the UK the MCNS is involved throughout the whole disease trajectory and patient pathway. Whilst other services such as oncology and palliative care will be involved as appropriate, the MCNS will usually remain a constant throughout the patient pathway. There appear to be few nurses in other countries working in dedicated mesothelioma roles. Anecdotally, nurses from Japan, Australia and the USA have expressed a desire to increase the number of nurses working in mesothelioma roles and replicate the UK model. However, countries without a single healthcare system may face a greater challenge developing a unified network of mesothelioma nurses.

The role of the MCNS at a local level is set out through a service level agreement between Mesothelioma UK and the host NHS organisation. Although the role may vary slightly, depending on the needs of the service, MCNSs are expected to incorporate four core duties into their role: patient care, information resources, service development and professional development. This aligns with the national framework of the four pillars of advanced practice: clinical practice, education, research and leadership (HEE, 2023).

Patient care

Patient care is at the heart of the MCNS role. Within the host NHS trust the MCNS is a key worker for a caseload of mesothelioma patients. The MCNS provides care and support across the patient pathway, using expert communication skills in explaining diagnoses, treatment options and preparing patients and families for end-of-life care (Taylor et al., 2019). Patients with mesothelioma are known to have a high symptom burden and therefore have significant palliative care needs. The MCNSs provide expert palliative care, which can mitigate the need for early referral to specialist palliative care services (Gardiner et al., 2022). Key MCNS roles include managing symptoms, providing psychological and emotional support, signposting to benefits and compensation advice, facilitating support groups, identifying the need for specialist palliative care involvement and supporting carers through bereavement (Gardiner et al., 2022). In addition to their local caseload the MCNS also accepts referrals from other teams within their region/Cancer Alliance, usually providing remote support by telephone or in person at support groups.

At a national level the MCNS provides expertise via the charity's support line. This is a free service for patients, carers and healthcare professionals to seek specialist advice and guidance on mesothelioma by telephone or email. These clinical duties set the MCNS role apart from most other cancer CNS roles which traditionally hold one caseload locally within their NHS organisation.

Skilled care coordination is important in improving the patient experience (Macmillan Cancer Support, 2017). This is essential in mesothelioma, due to the association with asbestos and resultant benefits and compensation needs. The MCNS provides vital signposting through networks with other services such as charitable organisations and support groups, in addition to specialist legal teams, who guide patients and families through the process of litigation. The MCNS builds and fosters effective working relationships with stakeholders in their region and across the UK to ensure patients receive specialist advice and support on all issues relating to mesothelioma. The MCNS is key to nurturing multiservice partnerships with charities and wider stakeholders enabling patients and carers to access and holistic care.

Information resources/evaluation

MCNSs contribute to local, regional and national datasets such as organisational patient data systems and the national mesothelioma audit (Royal College of Physicians, 2020). Mesothelioma UK datasets capture episodes of care such as symptom management, clinical trials and psychological support. This data gives valuable national and local insight as well as evidence on the breadth of the MCNS role.

As core members of lung or specialist mesothelioma multidisciplinary teams (MDT), the MCNS advocates for patients and provides clinical expertise in mesothelioma to the wider team. They keep abreast of all clinical trial opportunities via an app created by Mesothelioma UK (2021) to ensure patients are aware of opportunities and able to make informed decisions regarding participation. The app provides information about the nearest recruiting centres and trial entry requirements, ensuring treatment options for patients are optimised.

Service development/leadership

MCNSs participate in and often lead service development. They are engaged in clinical audit, patient experience and research, identifying, designing and completing their own research projects. The more senior MCNSs provide mentorship to junior colleagues. Regionally the MCNS is an expert voice within the Cancer Alliance, supporting other teams in the region to recognise the support needs of this patient. The MCNS supports national awareness events such as Action Mesothelioma Day, organising and facilitating activities within their area. Education delivery forms a large part of the role, delivering presentations at local, national and international events.

MCNSs also contribute to the development of the national Mesothelioma UK nursing service to improve patient care. One recent development was the introduction of the peritoneal MCNS (PMCNS) mentioned above. Peritoneal mesothelioma poses considerable challenges due to the rarity of the disease, such as lack of experienced healthcare professionals and access to specialist advice. This role was the first of its kind nationally, and to our knowledge, internationally (Mesothelioma UK, 2018). The PMCNS is based at the Peritoneal Malignancy Institute, host of the national peritoneal MDT that receives referrals from all four UK nations. They expertly guide patients, families and healthcare teams through diagnosis, treatment options and symptom management, ensuring geography is not a barrier to providing seamless specialist care. The PMCNS has developed new and innovative ways to connect patients for peer-to-peer support with a unique buddy system, organising and facilitating an online support group and a private Facebook group with over 400 members. The impact of the role has received national recognition, being awarded Oncology Nurse of the Year at the *British Journal of Nursing* awards in 2023.

Professional development

Professional development not only refers to the MCNSs' own continuing professional development, but also their contribution to the development of the wider team. When appointed, a MCNS will already be an experienced nurse, committed to personal and professional development. Once in post the MCNS identifies their own learning and development needs, with some undertaking additional training, in areas such as genomic medicine, leadership and palliative care.

In addition to developing and sharing relevant resources with patients and carers, they also share information with colleagues. In a recent research study, MCNSs reflected on the value of developing a collective knowledge base through sharing resources via the Mesothelioma UK network (Gardiner et al., 2022), highlighting the value of learning and educating others across the UK-wide community of MCNSs.

Evidence of the value of the MCNS role

Patients, carers and wider healthcare teams have a positive experience of the care provided by cancer CNSs. Recent research has identified the clear contribution of the CNS in relation to psychological support, education, symptom management, service coordination and patient satisfaction (Kerr et al., 2021). Furthermore, patients have reported that they highly value their relationship with their cancer CNS, particularly when that relationship starts early in the diagnosis of mesothelioma (Taylor et al, 2019). Having a named CNS has been associated with better experiences of care: being involved in treatment decisions, perceiving care as more coordinated, being treated with respect and dignity and reporting a positive overall experience (Alessy et al., 2021). Care by a CNS is also found to increase the uptake of anticancer treatments by patients with lung cancer and has been associated with increased survival rates (Stewart et al., 2018; Alessy et al., 2024).

The Mesothelioma UK MCNS model is widely regarded as the gold standard and one to which other rare cancer charities and other countries' healthcare systems could aspire to. Increased global collaboration through organisations such as the International Thoracic Oncology Forum (ITONF) and the International Mesothelioma Interest Group (iMig) have increased the visibility and impact of the MCNS role.

Threats to the CNS role in mesothelioma

The Mesothelioma UK CNS model is a modern nursing success story. Its remarkable success has been achieved with no financial support from the NHS, relying on charitable monies to fund the nursing posts. Unfortunately, this is also what makes it vulnerable. Without central financial support, the sustainability of MCNS posts can never be guaranteed. The Covid-19 pandemic and recent global instability that resulted in a cost-of-living crisis has seen charity funding reduce dramatically. This means that growth of the team been a considerable challenge as has maintaining continued funding for the existing posts. The contribution of MCNSs is not always visible to their organisations and Cancer Alliances.

Cancer service guidance in the UK such as the Getting It Right First Time (GIRFT) programme (NHS England, 2024), in addition to NICE guidelines, have ensured that CNSs are embedded as core members of every cancer team. For example, the NICE guidance for lung cancer (2024) states that "all cancer units/centres should have one or more trained lung cancer CNS". In addition, the British Thoracic Society guideline for the investigation and management of malignant pleural mesothelioma recommends that each MDT has a named CNS for pleural mesothelioma (Woolhouse et al., 2018). However, without a mesothelioma NICE guideline that specifically recommends a dedicated specialist CNS the future is less certain. Limited awareness of the unique needs of those affected by mesothelioma also means that patients and families may have to fit into services designed for a different group of patients (lung cancer) rather than receiving care which is specifically determined to meet their needs.

Not all patients with a mesothelioma diagnosis have access to a CNS. Worryingly, the 2020 National Mesothelioma Audit showed the number of patients who were assessed by a CNS in England was still falling short of target at only 70%, while the number who had a CNS present at diagnosis was even lower at 57% (Royal College of Physicians, 2020). The audit did not determine whether it was a lung CNS or MCNS involved in patient care; however, it is clear from this data that there are still significant gaps in access to specialist support.

The previous chapter highlighted the nihilism that exists in mesothelioma among some healthcare professionals. This can be explained by the rarity of the disease, the perceived futility and limitation of treatment and the misconception that this disease is dying out. Furthermore, mesothelioma suffers from a lack of exposure to the public eye. Many people will be aware of the four most common cancers in the UK due to regular awareness campaigns on mainstream and social media. However, fewer people are aware of the incidence of mesothelioma. This is despite the fact that the UK has the highest rate of this disease in the world. These factors may also mean that investing in mesothelioma services is not perceived to be of high importance to policymakers and service providers. This is evident in the current inequality of access to specialist care and support, with some areas of the UK continuing to lack access to a MCNS at all.

The cancer CNS workforce is vulnerable. Several reports have highlighted the need for increased investment to ensure its sustainability to meet the needs of future patients (Macmillan Cancer Support, 2017). Also, cancer nurse specialists are an ageing workforce, with almost 40% of nurses aged over 50 (Macmillan Cancer Support, 2017). There has long been concern that cancer specialist nurses are less valued at times when frontline services are under pressure, with reports of specialist nurses being asked to cover shifts on wards (Macmillan Cancer Support, 2017). This was especially evident during the Covid-19 pandemic when CNSs were pulled into frontline areas despite their own workload changing. One study showed that 40% of CNSs were required to cover wards and other clinical services (Hargreaves et al., 2022). CNSs experience "moral distress" at being unable to complete work and leaving some care undone (Taylor et al., 2021; Hargreaves et al., 2022; Gardiner et al., 2022). Whilst particularly prevalent during Covid-19, this is not a new problem, having been highlighted in the literature more than five years before the pandemic occurred (Leary et al., 2014). These pressures are known to contribute to healthcare staff leaving their jobs, therefore action needs to be taken to support the nursing workforce through targeted retention strategies (World Health Organisation, 2022).

IMPLICATIONS FOR POLICY/PRACTICE

Evidence has demonstrated how valuable MCNSs are to patient care and multidisciplinary teams, delivering quality care and enhancing patient outcomes (Alessy et al., 2024; Kerr et al., 2021; Taylor et al., 2019). It also highlights how vulnerable the MCNS workforce is in light of the current funding structure, a lack of policy standards for mesothelioma care and a lack of knowledge and recognition of the value of MCNSs. To ensure the sustainability and development of the MCNS workforce there must be an ongoing commitment from central NHS policymakers to address the issues identified (Alessy et al., 2021).

Growth in the CNS workforce has predominantly been in the most common cancers such as lung, breast, prostate and bowel. However approximately 50% of people with cancer are diagnosed with a rare or less common cancer. This prompts a question of whether there should be a government plan, in the UK and other nations, to ensure equitable access to expert CNS care and support for rare as well as more common cancers.

Further research into the unique needs of patients and families affected by rare cancers is vital to ensure appropriate services are designed and delivered. A deeper understanding of the rare cancer CNS workforce is vital to demonstrate to commissioning bodies that investment in these services is pivotal in achieving better patient outcomes. Reporting the impact of the MCNS role is essential in demonstrating to commissioning bodies that MCNS roles should be funded as core services.

Increasing the visibility of the MCNS role is necessary to embed it as an essential part of care for patients with mesothelioma. At a local level it is important that visibility and access to MCNS posts must be increased among lung cancer teams to ensure appropriate patients are referred and given equitable access to specialist support. In areas where no MCNS post exists lung cancer teams should ensure patients are signposted to Mesothelioma UK who can enable patients to find support networks in their area and identify treatment options and clinical trial opportunities which may be open to them.

Standardising roles and promoting career development pathways are also important in maximising the impact of CNSs for patients, increasing acceptance and role clarity for colleagues and enhancing retention and succession planning (HEE, 2023). Suggested strategies to enhance the wellbeing of CNSs include peer support through shared reflections, hybrid working and compassionate organisational support (Hargreaves et al., 2022).

Proving value and increasing the visibility of the MCNS workforce poses a significant challenge. Small charities such as Mesothelioma UK do not have the resources of other larger cancer charities to continue to fund MCNSs. The NHS has become reliant on charities to shoulder the hidden cost of care given by CNSs. However, charities are struggling to sustain this financial burden. This situation creates challenges and vulnerabilities for the CNS workforce, not just in mesothelioma but in other cancers and health conditions.

REFERENCES

Alessy, S.A., Davies, E., Rawlinson, J., Baker, M. & Lüchtenborg, M. (2024). Clinical nurse specialists and survival in patients with cancer: The UK National Cancer Experience Survey. *BMJ Supportive & Palliative Care*, 14(e1), pp. e1208–e1224. https://spcare.bmj.com/content/bmjspcare/14/e1/e1208.full.pdf

Alessy, S.A., Lüchtenborg, M., Rawlinson, J., Baker, M. & Davies, E.A. (2021). Being assigned a clinical nurse specialist is associated with better experiences of cancer care: English population-based study using the linked National cancer patient experience survey and cancer registration dataset. *European Journal of Cancer Care*, 30(6), p. e13490. https://onlinelibrary.wiley.com/doi/10.1111/ecc.13490

Barton, T.D., Bevan, L. & Mooney, G. (2012). Advanced nursing. Part 1: The development of advanced nursing roles. *Nursing Times*, 108(24), pp. 18–20. https://pubmed.ncbi.nlm.nih.gov/22774671/

Cannaby, A.M., Carter, V., Rolland, P., Finn, A. & Owen, J. (2020). The scope and variance of clinical nurse specialist job descriptions. *British Journal of Nursing*, 29(11), pp.606–611.

Cancer Research UK (2024). *Mesothelioma incidence statistics*. Available at: https://www.cancerresearchuk.org/health-professional/cancer-statistics/statistics-by-cancer-type/mesothelioma/incidence#heading-Zero

Castledine, G. (2002). The development of the role of the clinical nurse specialist in the UK. *British Journal of Nursing*, 11(7), pp. 506–508. https://www.magonlinelibrary.com/doi/epdf/10.12968/bjon.2002.11.7.10154

Gardiner, C., et al. (2022). Clinical nurse specialist role in providing generalist and specialist palliative care: A qualitative study of mesothelioma clinical nurse specialists. *Journal of Advanced Nursing*, 78(9). pp. 2973–2982. https://eprints.whiterose.ac.uk/186328/

Hargreaves, S., Gardiner, C., Taylor, B., Tod, A., Ejegi-Memeh, S., Fennmore, J., Clayton, K., Darlison, L. & Creech, L. (2022), Impact of Covid-19 on lung cancer and mesothelioma specialist nurses: A survey of experiences and perceptions. *European Journal of Oncology Nursing*. https://doi.org/10.1016/j.ejon.2022.102207

Health Education England (2023). Career pathway, core capabilities and education framework. ACCEND programme. Available at: https://www.hee.nhs.uk/sites/default/files/documents/ACCEND%20Career%20Pathway%2C%20Core%20Cancer%20Capabilities%20and%20Education%20Framework.pdf (Accessed: 21 August 2024)

Kerr, H., Donovan, M. & McSorley, O. (2021). Evaluation of the role of the Clinical Nurse Specialist in cancer care: An integrative literature review. *European Journal of Cancer Care*, 30(3). p. e13415. https://doi.org/10.1111/ecc.13415

Leary, A., Maclaine, K., Trevatt, P., Radford, M. & Punshon, G. (2017). Variation in job titles within the nursing workforce. *Journal of Clinical Nursing*, 26(23–24):4945–4950. doi: 10.1111/jocn.13985. PMID: 28880423. https://pubmed.ncbi.nlm.nih.gov/28880423/

Leary, A., White, J. & Yarnell, L., (2014). The work left undone. Understanding the challenge of providing holistic lung cancer nursing care in the UK. *European Journal of Oncology Nursing*, 18(1), pp. 23–28. https://www.ejoncologynursing.com/article/S1462-3889(13)00129-4/abstract

Macmillan Cancer Support (2017). *Cancer workforce in England*. Available at: https://www.macmillan.org.uk/_images/cancer-workforce-in-england-census-of-cancer-palliative-and-chemotheraphy-speciality-nurses-and-support-workers-2017_tcm9-325727.pdf

Mesothelioma UK (2018). First UK peritoneal mesothelioma clinical nurse specialist appointed. Available at: https://www.mesothelioma.uk.com/first-uk-peritoneal-mesothelioma-clinical-nurse-specialist-appointed/

Mesothelioma UK (2021). Clinical trials app launched. Available at: https://www.mesothelioma.uk.com/clinical-trials-app-launched/

Mesothelioma UK (2024). Our nurses. Available at: https://www.mesothelioma.uk.com/our-nurses/

NHS England (2024). *Best practice timed diagnostic cancer pathways. GIRFT cancer programme*. Available at: https://gettingitrightfirsttime.co.uk/wp-content/uploads/2024/03/BestPracticeTimedDiagnosticCancerPathwayssummary-guide-March-24-V3.pdf

NICE (2024). *Lung cancer: Diagnosis and management. NG122*. Available at: https://www.nice.org.uk/guidance/ng122

Public Health England (2020). *National Cancer Registration and Analysis Service (NCRAS)*. Available at: https://www.gov.uk/guidance/national-cancer-registration-and-analysis-service-ncras

Royal College of Physicians (2020). *National Mesothelioma Audit report 2020 (for the audit period 2016–18)*. London: RCP. https://www.mesothelioma.uk.com/downloads/national-mesothelioma-audit-2020/?wpdmdl=15399

Stewart, I., Khakwani, A., Hubbard, R.B., Beckett, P., Borthwick, D., Tod, A., Leary, A. & Tata, L.J. (2018). Are working practices of lung cancer nurse specialists associated with variation in peoples' receipt of anticancer therapy? *Lung Cancer*, 123, pp.160–165. https://www.lungcancerjournal.info/article/S0169-5002(18)30482-3/fulltext

Taylor, B.H., et al. (2021). Effects of the COVID-19 pandemic on people with mesothelioma and their carers. *Cancer Nursing Practice*. https://doi.org/10.7748/cnp.2021.e1773

Taylor, B.H., Warnock, C. & Tod, A. (2019). Communication of a mesothelioma diagnosis: Developing recommendations to improve the patient experience. *BMJ Open Respiratory Research*, 6, p. e000413. https://doi.org/10.1136/bmjresp-2019-000413

Woolhouse, I., et al. (2018). British Thoracic Society guideline for the investigation and management of malignant pleural mesothelioma. *Thorax*, 73, p. i1–i30. https://thorax.bmj.com/content/73/Suppl_1/i1

World Health Organisation (2022). *Health and care workforce in Europe: Time to act*. Copenhagen: WHO Regional Office for Europe.

Chapter 4
The road to diagnosis

Bethany Taylor and Angela Tod

OVERVIEW

Both receiving and giving a cancer diagnosis is challenging and distressing. There are complexities associated with a diagnosis of mesothelioma (Ball et al., 2016). These include coming to terms with its cause and short prognosis as well as understanding the disease itself, treatment options and legal and financial implications.

Mesothelioma is almost exclusively caused by exposure to asbestos. The long period of time from asbestos exposure to disease (15–45 years) can amplify the struggle to understand the diagnosis. Thankfully, the treatment and trials landscape is improving. However, this can add to the already immense volume of information for patients and families to process. Mesothelioma is considered an industrial disease which brings with it financial and legal implications. This introduces further dimensions to the experience of patients and families at a time when they are already coming to terms with a mesothelioma diagnosis and what this means for them.

This chapter presents information on the diagnostic journey and the experiences of patients and their families at the time surrounding diagnosis. Presenting symptoms and diagnostic pathways, for both pleural and peritoneal mesothelioma, will be considered. This chapter will focus on the time when a mesothelioma diagnosis is given and the time following this when patients and families are processing the information.

The chapter aims to promote understanding of the experience of receiving a mesothelioma diagnosis from the perspectives of patients and their families, and to help healthcare professionals understand the importance of communicating a mesothelioma diagnosis well. This chapter will close by presenting key messages and recommendations for practice relating to communicating a diagnosis of mesothelioma.

DOI: 10.4324/9781032631318-4

THE EVIDENCE

Understanding of the challenges of receiving a mesothelioma diagnosis were generated by the Receiving a Diagnosis of Mesothelioma (RADIO Meso) study. Findings from RADIO Meso will be drawn upon in this chapter, alongside other research concerning the diagnostic experiences of specific groups, including people who were exposed in occupations not traditionally associated with asbestos exposure (including education and healthcare) and people with the rarer peritoneal mesothelioma.

RADIO Meso aimed to identify ways to improve the patient and family carer experience of receiving a diagnosis of mesothelioma and to generate evidence-based recommendations for practice. Six patients, nine family members and 16 healthcare professionals involved in communicating a diagnosis of mesothelioma were interviewed about their experiences. Two focus groups took place with 27 patients and 15 mesothelioma clinical nurse specialists. More details about this study are available at https://www.sheffield.ac.uk/murc/our-research/radio-meso and in Taylor et al.'s published article (2019).

The long, winding road to diagnosis

Evidence suggests that the route to receiving a diagnosis of this rare cancer can be complex and long (Taylor et al., 2019; Westbrook et al., 2025). The main symptoms of pleural mesothelioma are shortness of breath, chest pain, cough, sweating, loss of appetite, weight loss and fatigue. For peritoneal mesothelioma the main symptoms are abdominal pain and swelling, constipation or diarrhoea, feeling or being sick, loss of appetite, weight loss, sweating and fatigue. The symptoms people experience prior to receiving a diagnosis vary considerably. The nature of many of these symptoms means they can be described as vague or attributed to other conditions. This can delay patients from seeking advice because the symptoms are easily explained away or anticipated to pass with time.

Often the route to being diagnosed with mesothelioma begins with a visit to a GP when symptoms persist. For some pleural mesothelioma patients, their first contact with a healthcare professional is in an Accident and Emergency department due to breathlessness caused by a build-up of fluid on their lungs (pleural effusion). Wherever the patient presents with symptoms, they will be sent immediately or referred for tests that may include x-rays, ultrasound or CT scans. After initial imaging and control of immediate debilitating symptoms, referral for a biopsy will be made as tissue confirmation is essential prior to treatment.

The recommendation is that biopsy results will be discussed at a multidisciplinary team (MDT) meeting and where possible a specialist mesothelioma MDT. The rare nature of mesothelioma means that accessing a mesothelioma MDT can be difficult. If a mesothelioma diagnosis is confirmed, then a treatment plan will be considered. Although it sounds straightforward, reaching a diagnosis can be long and onerous. For example, with peritoneal mesothelioma, the diagnostic period is linked to great uncertainty and delays (Lond et al., 2024). A recent survey of 47 patients reported an average of 321 days between first experiencing symptoms and receiving an accurate diagnosis (Westbrook et al., 2025). Another survey of over 500 mesothelioma patients found that 25% visited their GP three or more times before being referred to the hospital for further tests (Mesothelioma UK, 2020).

The long diagnostic pathway for many patients is partly due to the non-specific symptoms experienced but also due to the rarity of mesothelioma which means it is unlikely that a GP will initially consider a diagnosis of mesothelioma. This is particularly the case if a person is not aware of their asbestos exposure. A GP may ask the question *"Have you ever worked with asbestos?"* or ask about a patient's previous occupation. The index of suspicion for mesothelioma is understandably higher when a person has worked in an industry associated with asbestos exposure, such as construction, shipbuilding or mining. Increasingly, people are being exposed to asbestos in environments built or renovated prior to the asbestos ban that still contain asbestos. These people are often unaware of their exposure. Their occupational history is unlikely to be flagged as high risk so people may face additional delays in reaching their diagnosis.

A GP is likely to rule out other potential causes of symptoms first and this can take time. Abdominal symptoms experienced by peritoneal mesothelioma patients mean that they are often referred to gynaecology or colorectal speciality teams who may have limited experience of mesothelioma. Patients may undergo tests and procedures that will not detect mesothelioma and therefore come back negative. This can cause uncertainty and frustration for people who desperately want reassurance but also an explanation and treatment for the persisting symptoms. This is illustrated by the following experience of someone whose partner developed mesothelioma after asbestos exposure in healthcare:

> *[We] had consultants that wouldn't accept that she wasn't suffering from something normal. Mesothelioma should be sort of kept at the back of everybody's mind, I think. It's not the first port of call, but when you've got something strange and you don't know what it is you can't rule it out. And the consultant I think said it couldn't be some things because she hadn't worked in industry.*
>
> (Allmark et al., 2020, p. 15)

A diagnosis can be further complicated if a person is incorrectly diagnosed with other conditions before receiving a mesothelioma diagnosis. Examples for pleural mesothelioma include lung cancer, chest infection, pleural plaques and exacerbation of pre-existing conditions such as COPD. For peritoneal mesothelioma these include ovarian cancer, endometriosis and a cancer of unknown primary (Westbrook et al., 2025).

Receiving the news

Receiving a diagnosis of mesothelioma is life changing, it has a long-lasting impact on patients and families. Sadly, a survey of over 500 mesothelioma patients reported that 27% felt that their diagnosis could have been given more sensitively (Mesothelioma UK, 2020). In a research study of 47 peritoneal patients, 70% said the diagnosis was understandable and 62% said their diagnosis was given in a sensitive way (Westbrook et al., 2025). These findings show that there is room for improvement when communicating a diagnosis of mesothelioma but that there are also examples of good practice to learn from, as demonstrated here: *"She said it with, again, such compassion… I felt she was totally looking after me, my interests, not anything else"* (Westbrook et al., 2025).

A supportive environment is important when receiving this incredibly challenging diagnosis. Ideally, the room should be quiet and private with sufficient seating for everyone to feel comfortable. Feeling overheard or being disturbed in a busy clinic environment can make this communication more difficult for all involved. One family member of someone with mesothelioma described their experience: *"We were just took in a small little room, I don't even think there was enough chairs for us to sit on, and told it's mesothelioma, which we couldn't even say, let alone know what it was"* (Taylor et al., 2019, p. 8).

The way that information is communicated is as significant as the words used. Communication skills valued by patients and their families include the ability to communicate in a warm, inclusive and respectful way. Allocating appropriate time and creating a sense of time are also essential to good communication of a mesothelioma diagnosis. If a diagnosis is delivered poorly, it can intensify distress and lead to lasting confusion and resentment (Warnock, 2014; Warnock et al., 2010).

When receiving a diagnosis, people vary tremendously in the amount of information they want to know and can take on board. Although some patients and their family members are keen to seek as much information as possible, others can feel overloaded and burdened with information. Use of unnecessary medical terms and technical language can make receiving a diagnosis more challenging and isolating, sometimes raising more questions than are answered. The quote from a patient below illustrates how some people can feel overwhelmed by the shock of their diagnosis:

> *I certainly didn't understand mesothelioma at all really… although I was going to say I looked it up on the internet, initially I don't think I did anything because I was a little bit taken aback and there was quite a bit of shock and upset and we didn't know really what to do, if the truth is known. And that's unusual for me because I would normally grasp it right away and be in control of it, but I wasn't.*
>
> (Taylor et al., 2018, p. 8)

There are a growing number of treatments, enabling some people with mesothelioma to live longer. The decision to have treatment and, if so, which treatment is complex. Treatments carry significant side effects and can sadly not yet provide a cure. At diagnosis, some patients can feel relatively well and active so may be advised to "watch and wait" for their symptoms to develop further before seeking treatment. This uncertainty can be difficult for people seeking a clear treatment pathway. In some cases, people may also be given information about clinical trials as a possible treatment option at the time of diagnosis. This opens a whole new realm of information to understand as many patients are not familiar with clinical trials and concepts such as randomisation which can be difficult to grasp. Patients may feel disappointed by the uncertainty and expect healthcare professionals to know what treatment is best for them (this is discussed further in Chapter 5 (treatment options and experiences) and Chapter 8 (barriers and facilitators to clinical trial participation)).

A mesothelioma diagnosis makes it necessary for the individual and their family to navigate the various services and systems with a rare cancer. This includes the NHS, the benefits system and possibly the legal system. Meanwhile, they are likely to be experiencing troublesome symptoms. Some, due to the poor prognosis, have a limited time available to do this.

The financial and legal aspects of a mesothelioma diagnosis add another layer of information for patients and families to absorb and are unique to mesothelioma. There is variation and much discussion over when it is best to inform people that 1) they may be eligible to seek compensation following their exposure to asbestos and 2) that an investigation by a coroner (Procurator Fiscal in Scotland) will be required after death due to the industrial nature of the disease. The diagnostic appointment may not be the appropriate time to share information about these two aspects, yet there are reasons why it is important that patients and families are informed in a timely manner. A successful compensation claim cannot only ease the financial pressures on the family but also open doors to non-NHS-funded treatments which may improve quality and length of life. These claims can take time so there is some sense of urgency in starting this process. Regarding coroner involvement, if families are not prepared this can cause additional emotional trauma and stress (Taylor et al., 2024.)

The prognosis

One of the most challenging aspects of a mesothelioma diagnosis is the impact that this has on a person's life expectancy. Some patients and families instinctively ask '*How long do I/they have left?*' but may not be equipped to hear the response. Others are fully aware that they do not wish to know the answer to this question. There may be variation within families regarding information preferences. The person with mesothelioma, and their family, should be given the opportunity to say whether they want a discussion about prognosis. This area of practice requires great sensitivity and experience. It is helpful to check with people what they have already been told before giving new information, especially regarding prognosis.

It is worth noting here that when healthcare professionals are asked about prognosis, it is incredibly difficult to answer accurately. Prognosis is influenced by factors such as stage of the disease at diagnosis, cell type, overall health and response to treatment. Predicting how factors will interact and affect an individual's prognosis is complex. Further to this, with mesothelioma being a rare disease, data to predict outcomes is limited. While it is of course understandable for people to ask this question and to look to healthcare professionals for certainty and knowledge, there sadly remains much uncertainty with mesothelioma and this adds to the distress patients and their families feel.

The impact of receiving a diagnosis of mesothelioma

Receiving a diagnosis of mesothelioma has a profound impact on the mental health and wellbeing of patients and their families. Receiving any cancer diagnosis is incredibly distressing. However, there is evidence to suggest that the nature of mesothelioma, including its high symptom burden, preventable and unjust cause, incurability and associated financial and legal implications cause unique mental health and wellbeing impacts (Ejegi-Memeh et al., 2022; Sherborne et al., 2020). Research indicates that a mesothelioma diagnosis can cause trauma, depression and anxiety for patients and their family members (Bonafede et al., 2022; Sherborne et al., 2020; Ejegi-Memeh et al., 2022; Sherborne et al., 2024). Acknowledging the magnitude of the diagnosis on family members, as well as patients, and the impact on them and their lives is very important. The mental health and wellbeing impact of a mesothelioma diagnosis is considered in more depth in Chapter 13.

For those who were unaware of their asbestos exposure, the shock and devastation of receiving a mesothelioma diagnosis can be exacerbated (Taylor et al., 2022). This lack of awareness adds another layer of complexity to comprehend. Regardless of whether they knew about the exposure, patients and their families can feel immense anger and frustration. Mesothelioma is a preventable cancer, and there is a strong sense of injustice that people's lives have been irrevocably altered by asbestos exposure – an exposure they were either unaware of or not adequately warned about. One patient exposed to asbestos working as a health professional said: "'*I think personally now, it's ironic, that I've dedicated 44 years of my life, and you know, that dedication is what's killing me now. It's ironic really.*' Interview with a health professional with mesothelioma" (Allmark et al., 2020, p. 16).

Alongside the negative impacts of a mesothelioma diagnosis, some patients and family members report positive impacts as well (Sherborne et al., 2020; 2024; Ejegi-Memeh et al., 2024). These can include living life with a sense of freedom, a greater appreciation for the joy in every day and growing as a person.

Personalising the diagnosis and finding hope

This chapter has so far demonstrated that there is not a "one size fits all" approach to communicating a mesothelioma diagnosis. The information and support that patients and their families require varies, as does the pace at which they are ready to process it. Making sense of the diagnosis often includes coming to terms with the personal implications for the person with mesothelioma and their loved ones.

Some people find comfort in separating themselves from the statistics. This is particularly the case for women and younger patients who may not feel represented in the average statistics because the majority are men (83%) and are older (60% of deaths from mesothelioma are over 75). It is also challenging for those who are physically fit at diagnosis with no other health issues. There are a growing number of people living longer with mesothelioma. As mentioned above, it is difficult to give an accurate prognosis to individuals, despite survival statistics. Potential reasons for this include the changing demographic of mesothelioma patients, with more people being diagnosed at a younger age and the improving treatment landscape. There are people who survive and live with mesothelioma for a long time, despite being told at diagnosis that they have months to live (Johnson et al., 2022). Many people find hope in such survival stories.

In the RADIO Meso study, patients and family members talked about how important it was for health professionals to be direct and honest about their diagnosis but to balance this with hope. Hope can come from symptom management, new treatment options and setting goals. Below, the wife of a patient talks about how she lives in hope following her husband's diagnosis:

> *And so, you know, we live in hope. [My husband] is 68, we want to get him to at least 70, so... we're setting little goals out for ourselves all the time, doing things and trying to enjoy things that we'd never done before – like go and visit a test match... doing nice things, creating magical memories I've been calling it. Everywhere we go, taking pictures and spending more time with our grandchildren, spending more time with [my husband's] brother and my family.*
>
> (Taylor et al., 2018, p. 17)

Receiving a diagnosis is a process, not an event

While a diagnosis of mesothelioma may be confirmed at a specific appointment, such as an out-patient clinic or on a ward, communicating the diagnosis and the associated information is a process that happens over time. This was a key finding from the RADIO Meso study. The process starts when mesothelioma is first suspected and continues as people start to understand their diagnosis and its many implications. If a diagnosis is to be communicated well, this process should provide continuity and consistency in terms of who the patient and family see, and what is said to them. The importance of viewing breaking bad news as a process is reinforced by Warnock et al. (2010; Warnock, 2014).

Sources of support when a person has received a mesothelioma diagnosis

Once a person and their family receive a mesothelioma diagnosis, they are thrust into navigating services to try and find out who to contact, when, why and how. A range of professionals and services are involved in providing information and support. This is partly due to the complexity of a mesothelioma diagnosis. Some of these key support roles are now described:

Clinical nurse specialists. Mesothelioma or lung cancer nurse specialists provide essential support and care and are a key point of contact for patients (see Chapter 3 for more information on the role of CNSs). A CNS is usually the person providing follow-up care once somebody has been given their diagnosis. CNSs help to facilitate communication across the diagnostic pathway and between the MDT members, promoting continuity and consistency, for example, explaining what is happening and why regarding diagnostic procedures, tests and appointments and tracking progress through these.

Asbestos Support Groups (ASGs). In the UK these groups are often best placed to give information and support families to complete the paperwork required to access benefits they are entitled to and initial information about seeking compensation.

Benefits advice services. There are various organisations providing benefits advice. Some focus on cancer, for example, Macmillan-funded advisors, others are more generic, such as the Citizens Advice Bureau. For UK military veterans benefits advice and support is available from Veterans UK. Provision of benefits advice may vary across UK regions but, where available, they can provide an invaluable source of support and information.

Legal firms specialising in mesothelioma help patients navigate the complex legal system and secure compensation for the harm caused by asbestos exposure, holding their hands throughout this process.

Mesothelioma UK is a national charity dedicated to supporting people affected by mesothelioma. They fund or part fund a network of mesothelioma CNSs. They also provide an abundance of information and support for patients, families and professionals concerning all aspects of a mesothelioma diagnosis, including a helpline.

People affected by mesothelioma can find great comfort and helpful information from connecting with other patients and families, in addition to professional sources of support. With mesothelioma being a rare cancer, this can be difficult. People tend to connect on the growing social media community or through attending face-to-face or virtual support group meetings hosted by Mesothelioma UK or ASGs.

IMPLICATIONS FOR POLICY/PRACTICE

Receiving a diagnosis of mesothelioma is incredibly challenging and heartbreaking, but it can be communicated effectively and supportively. The RADIO Meso study findings have provided an evidence base for a set of recommendations to guide healthcare professionals in delivering a mesothelioma diagnosis. These "Ten Top Tips" have been endorsed by Mesothelioma UK and are summarised below. Further information about how to implement these and more detail about the RADIO Meso study can be found in the report (Taylor et al., 2018).

Ten top tips when communicating a mesothelioma diagnosis:

1   Provide consistency and continuity in terms of who the patients sees and what is said.
2   Involve the clinical nurse specialist throughout, starting as early as possible in the diagnostic pathway.
3   Ensure that staff involved in communicating a diagnosis of mesothelioma have specialist knowledge and training in mesothelioma as well as communication skills. Training should be ongoing with access to regular updates.
4   Be patient-centred when communicating a diagnosis. Take cues from the patient and family in balancing what information to give and when. Use language that is easy to understand. Don't just rely on written information and booklets.
5   Ensure the patient feels they have been allocated enough time.
6   Provide a quiet and private environment
7   Make the patient feel like the most important person in the room, and at the centre of the communication process
8   Be direct and honest whilst maintaining hope where possible, for example, by providing information about appropriate treatments, symptom management and trials.
9   Use available expertise and resources. No single clinician should carry the responsibility of communicating a diagnosis on their own. Best practice is often from partnership working with difficult services and quality resources.
10   Prepare and plan as a team before communicating a diagnosis of mesothelioma. This should include the communication of a plan for ongoing management and treatment to the patient and family carer.

It is important to note that healthcare staff often work within resource constraints such as limited time, challenging environments and insufficient staffing. These constraints can sometimes impact their ability to achieve best practice. These recommendations are aspirational and summarise factors that can enable effective communication. They may also be useful in other scenarios where bad news needs to be communicated, such as informing patients that they are not eligible for a particular treatment or clinical trial in which they had invested hope.

IMPLICATIONS FOR POLICY/PRACTICE

One of the challenges in practice is disseminating these recommendations to people who don't work with mesothelioma patients regularly. With mesothelioma being a rare cancer, many healthcare professionals do not have experience of caring for these patients. This generates inequitable access to specialist care and support for patients which impacts on their experience and outcomes.

In a study investigating the pathway for people with peritoneal mesothelioma (Westbrook et al., 2025), healthcare professional participants recognised that the majority of their knowledge was based on pleural mesothelioma as these patients formed the largest part of their clinical caseload. This highlights the importance of discussing every patient at an MDT. At the time of writing, there is a national MDT for people with peritoneal mesothelioma. However, there is a challenge in raising awareness of this so that people are referred early to aid diagnosis and treatment decisions.

Consistent with changing demographics and evolving treatment/trial landscapes, research is required to inform approaches to discussing prognosis effectively. There is also space for research to explore the experiences of young people and children affected by a mesothelioma diagnosis (for example, if their parents are diagnosed).

Receiving a diagnosis of mesothelioma is undeniably devastating. While the harsh reality cannot be softened, delivering the diagnosis with kindness and humility can greatly enhance the experience for patients and their families. Each patient has their own story to tell about receiving such news. Healthcare professionals cannot change the diagnosis, but they can ensure that each patient's story is one of support and compassion.

REFERENCES

Allmark, P., Tod, A.M. & Darlison, L. (2020). *MAGS: The Healthcare Staff Mesothelioma Asbestos Guidance Study*. Available at: https://www.mesothelioma.uk.com/past-research-projects/#mags (Accessed: 16 August 2024)

Ball, H., Moore, S. & Leary, A. (2016). A systematic literature review comparing the psychological care needs of patients with mesothelioma and advanced lung cancer. *European Journal of Oncology Nursing*, 25, pp. 62–67. https://doi.org/10.1016/j.ejon.2016.09.007

Bonafede, M., et al. (2022). Preliminary validation of a questionnaire assessing psychological distress in caregivers of patients with malignant mesothelioma: Mesothelioma Psychological Distress Tool – Caregivers. *Psycho-Oncology*, 31(1), pp. 122–129. https://doi.org/10.1002/pon.5789

Ejegi-Memeh, S., et al. (2022). Patients' and informal carers' experience of living with mesothelioma: a systematic rapid review and synthesis of the literature. *European Journal of Oncology Nursing*, 58(102122). https://doi.org/10.1016/j.ejon.2022.102122

Ejegi-Memeh, S., et al. (2024). Mental health and wellbeing in mesothelioma: A qualitative study exploring what helps the wellbeing of those living with this illness and their informal carers. *European Journal of Oncology Nursing*, 70 (102572). https://doi.org/10.1016/j.ejon.2024.102572

Johnson, M., Allmark, P. & Tod A. (2022) Living beyond expectations: A qualitative study into the experience of long-term survivors with pleural mesothelioma and their carers. *BMJ Open Respiratory Research*, 9(1). https://doi.org/10.1136/bmjresp-2022-001252

Lond, B., Apps, L., Quincey, K. & Williamson, I. (2024). The psychological impact of living with peritoneal mesothelioma: An interpretative phenomenological analysis. *Journal of Health Psychology*. https://doi.org/10.1177/13591053241298932

Mesothelioma UK. (2020) *Mesothelioma Outcomes, Research and Experience Survey (MORE) April 2020*. Available at: https://mesothelioma.uk.com/wp-content/uploads/dlm_uploads/2021/02/More-Report-2020-Final-singles.pdf (Accessed: November 2024)

Sherborne, V. et al. (2020) What are the psychological effects of mesothelioma on patients and their carers? A scoping review. *Psycho-Oncology*, 29(10), pp. 1464–11473. https://doi.org/10.1002/pon.5454

Sherborne, V., et al. (2024) The mental health and well-being implications of a mesothelioma diagnosis: A mixed methods study. *European Journal of Oncology Nursing*, 70 (102545). https://doi.org/10.1016/j.ejon.2024.102545

Taylor, B., et al. (2024). 68 How do family members experience coroner or procurator fiscal involvement following a mesothelioma death? *Lung Cancer*, 190 (107629). https://doi.org/10.1016/j.lungcan.2024.107629

Taylor, B., Allmark, P., Tod, A. (2022) The experiences of presentation, diagnosis, treatment and care for school-based education workers with mesothelioma: A scoping review. *International Journal of Nursing Health Care Research*, 5(1342). https://doi.org/10.29011/2688-9501.101342

Taylor, B., Tod, A., Stanley, H., Ball, H. & Warnock, C. (2018). Communicating a diagnosis of mesothelioma: Findings and Recommendations from the Radio Meso study. Final report. Available at: https://www.sheffield.ac.uk/murc/our-research/radio-meso

Taylor, B., Warnock, C. & Tod, A. (2019). Communication of a mesothelioma diagnosis: Developing recommendations to improve the patient experience. *BMJ Open Respiratory Research*, 6(1), e000413. https://doi.org/10.1136/bmjresp-2019-000413

Warnock, C. (2014). Breaking bad news: Issues relating to nursing practice. *Nursing Standard*, 28(45), pp. 51–58. https://doi.org/10.7748/ns.28.45.51.e8935

Warnock, C., et al. (2010). Breaking bad news in inpatient clinical settings: Role of the nurse. *Journal of Advanced Nursing*, 66(7), pp. 1543–1555. https://doi.org/10.1111/j.1365-2648.2010.05325.x

Westbrook, S., et al. (2025). Variation in the diagnostic and treatment pathway in peritoneal mesothelioma: A mixed-methods study in the United Kingdom. *European Journal of Cancer Care*, 8875835. https://doi.org/10.1155/ecc/8875835

Chapter 5

Treatment experiences

Anna Bibby, Anna Morley and Clare Warnock

OVERVIEW

When considering treatment options for mesothelioma, it is important to remain mindful of the intended treatment goals. Therapeutic aims may include palliation of symptom, extension of life expectancy or optimisation of quality of life (QoL). Although there are cases of long-term survival with mesothelioma, treatment is not curative (Royal College of Physicians, 2020). Hence, all decisions relating to mesothelioma treatment need to balance individual patient benefit against the risk of complications or side effects. For some, this may include a "watchful waiting" or active surveillance approach rather than immediately starting oncological treatment. A key component of this decision-making is patients' experiences of the different treatment modalities, which this chapter aims to summarise.

THE EVIDENCE

Experiences of receiving treatment: Standard care

Patients' experiences of treatment for mesothelioma vary considerably. Different experiences have been described by patients with regards to access to treatment, incidence and severity of side effects and treatment outcomes (Johnson et al., 2022; Watts et al., 2024). This section provides an overview of the range of experiences and the potential physical, emotional and social impacts on patients.

The current standard of care for mesothelioma is systemic anticancer therapy, specifically chemotherapy or immunotherapy, which has been shown to help people live longer with mesothelioma. However, it is unclear whether systemic anticancer treatment needs to be started immediately after diagnosis, and so some people (often those who feel well and are not experiencing symptoms from their mesothelioma)

DOI: 10.4324/9781032631318-5

choose to delay treatment until there is evidence of disease progression or until symptoms start to bother them. This "watchful waiting" approach is likely to maximise quality of life, with no obvious negative impact on length of life (Schmid et al., 2024).

Drug treatment options

Treatment options for mesothelioma have progressed significantly in recent years. Historically, chemotherapy using the combination of pemetrexed and either cisplatin or carboplatin was the standard of care. This regimen offers a survival benefit of 2.8 months compared with single-agent chemotherapy (Vogelzang et al., 2003). In the past decade, several new systemic treatment approaches have been shown to have benefit in pleural mesothelioma. These include first-line combination immunotherapy with nivolumab and ipilimumab, the new standard of care in most countries (Baas et al., 2021), the addition of the anti-angiogenesis agent bevacizumab to front-line chemotherapy (Zalcman et al., 2016) and the use of arginine depletion agents in non-epithelioid subtypes (Szlosarek et al., 2024). Unfortunately, many of the trials did not include patients with peritoneal disease, with the exception of the CONFIRM trial, which supported the use of single-agent nivolumab for people with pleural or peritoneal disease who have relapsed following initial chemotherapy (Fennell et al., 2021). In a recent study, Lond et al. (2024) indicated that the lack or research and knowledge of peritoneal disease can leave patients feeling a sense of isolation and feeling unsupported.

The use of these newer systemic anticancer agents is supported by robust randomised trial evidence demonstrating clear and meaningful survival benefits and, where measured, no detrimental impact on QoL. However, the drugs do have side effects, and patients should be counselled about these during the decision-making process. Happily, there is currently a healthy level of mesothelioma clinical trial activity. This will lead to new understanding of what drives mesothelioma and how to treat it.

Surgical treatment options

Mesothelioma can be difficult to diagnose. For most people, the first line of investigations includes a biopsy, done either under image guidance or medical thoracoscopy (for pleural disease). However, if these initial tests do not achieve a confirmed diagnosis, surgical biopsy may be needed. For pleural disease, this will take the form of a VATS (video-assisted thoracic surgery) biopsy, whilst for people with peritoneal mesothelioma a laparoscopy may be required.

Patients with pleural mesothelioma who require a surgical biopsy may benefit from having surgical pleurodesis (a procedure to stick the lining of the lung to the chest wall and prevent fluid build-up) at the same time. However, if surgery is not required for diagnostic purposes, medical pleurodesis with talc via a chest drain is preferable, as it is less invasive and associated with fewer complications (Rintoul et al., 2014). See below for more detail about managing fluid build-up.

The role of surgery in the treatment of pleural mesothelioma is a controversial area. Historically, surgical options for pleural mesothelioma ranged from the most aggressive extra-pleural pneumonectomy (EPP), where the affected lung, visceral and parietal pleura, diaphragm and pericardium are resected, to the less invasive debulking partial pleurectomy (PP) procedure, where tumour is stripped from the visible visceral and parietal pleura, but the lung, mediastinal pleural surfaces and diaphragm/pericardium are left untouched. Randomised controlled clinical trials do not support the use of either operation in mesothelioma, showing surgery to be associated with more complications, longer hospital stays, reduced quality of life and, for EPP, more deaths compared with standard, non-surgical treatment (Treasure et al., 2011; Rintoul et al., 2014).

A question remains about whether partial pleurectomy may be useful in non-expansile or "trapped" lung, where the mesothelioma tumour has encased the lung and is preventing it from expanding. A recent trial aiming to investigate this did not manage to recruit enough patients, perhaps because this condition tends to be associated with more advanced disease.

More recently, the MARS2 trial investigated the role of the remaining "middle ground" operation: extended pleurectomy decortication (EP/D), where the entire visceral and parietal pleura are removed, alongside the pericardium and diaphragm, but the lung is left in situ. MARS2 found EP/D (performed after two cycles of induction chemotherapy) caused more harm, in the form of increased adverse events, more deaths, shorter overall survival and reduced quality of life, compared with chemotherapy alone (Lim et al., 2024). Response to this well-conducted, multicentre randomised trial has been polarised, with some clinicians maintaining that there is still a role for surgery in carefully selected cases (Grosso et al., 2024). However, most international guidelines do not recommend surgery as routine treatment for pleural mesothelioma, unless in the context of a clinical trial (Woolhouse et al., 2018; Scherpereel et al., 2020).

In peritoneal disease, surgery to remove all visible tumour from the abdomen is sometimes performed and is often followed by hyperthermic intraperitoneal chemotherapy (HIPEC – where the abdomen is washed with heated chemotherapy at the end of the operation, to treat any cancer cells remaining). The evidence for this procedure is limited, and the procedure may not be suitable for everyone, hence, in the UK, it is only performed at the specialist national peritoneal mesothelioma centre in

Basingstoke. Recent evidence revealed that women with peritoneal mesothelioma can experience a loss of femininity and fertility due to abdominal swelling pre-surgery and scarring, and medically induced menopause following surgery (Lond et al., 2024)

Radiotherapy options

Radiotherapy can provide symptomatic relief from pain associated with mesothelioma, although response to treatment varies (Macleod et al., 2014). In situations where mesothelioma tumour has spread down the tract of previous interventional procedures, known as tract metastases, and is causing pain, targeted radiotherapy may alleviate symptoms (Clive et al., 2016; Bayman et al., 2019). However, prophylactic radiotherapy delivered immediately after procedures are performed to prevent tract metastases appearing is not necessary, nor recommended (Clive et al., 2016; Woolhouse et al., 2018; Bayman et al., 2019).

The treatment landscape for mesothelioma remains dynamic, with several innovative anticancer approaches currently under investigation in clinical trials. An example of a current experimental treatment is proton beam therapy, a type of high-energy radiotherapy that is able to target tumours very precisely, causing less impact to surrounding tissues. Considerations around clinical trials are covered in more detail in Chapter 8.

Chemotherapy

In qualitative research studies of mesothelioma, patients report variation in the problems they encountered with some experiencing considerable challenges, such as prolonged fatigue and nausea (Johnson et al., 2022) while others experience fewer side effects. There are no detailed studies exploring the incidence and severity of chemotherapy side effects among mesothelioma patients. However, a self-reported survey of patients with advanced lung cancer treated with cisplatin/carboplatin and pemetrexed found the most commonly experienced problems included fatigue, decreased appetite, taste changes, mucositis, constipation/diarrhoea and rash (Visser et al., 2018). The incidence and severity of these side effects varied between patients. Other serious potential side effects associated with this regimen include neutropenic sepsis, renal damage and peripheral neuropathy.

Immunotherapy

The introduction of immunotherapy as a treatment for mesothelioma has been viewed as a positive advance. However, it should be noted that variation exists in outcomes, with some patients having a limited response while others have prolonged disease control (Wiesenthal et al., 2018). This is associated, in some cases, with considerable improvements in disease-related symptoms and quality of life (Park et al., 2020). A systematic review of qualitative studies exploring patient experience of immunotherapy found that patients who had received chemotherapy and immunotherapy tended to view immunotherapy more favourably as it was felt to have less toxicities with some patients feeling comparatively well between treatments (Watts et al., 2024).

The side effects of immunotherapy and chemotherapy are very different in terms of their nature, timing, duration and management (Wiesenthal et al., 2018). Immunotherapy side effects, called immune-related adverse events (IRAEs), can potentially affect any tissue in the body, but are most commonly seen in gastrointestinal, skin, endocrine, musculoskeletal, respiratory, liver and renal systems (Jamieson et al., 2020). They may occur weeks or months into treatment and, in some cases, can persist for months to years following treatment completion (Ala-Leppilami et al., 2020). However, the incidence and severity of IRAEs varies considerably between patients with many experiencing minimal to moderate and short-term effects while a smaller number face severe, potentially long-lasting and, in rare cases, life-threatening IRAEs (Jamieson et al., 2020). In addition, considerable differences exist in individual symptom experience in terms of when they occur over the course of treatment, their duration, severity, impact on daily life and long-term effects (Park et al., 2020, Ala-Leppilami et al., 2020).

The impact of immunotherapy treatment extends beyond physical sequelae. Patients receiving immunotherapy have described their experience as living in a permanent state of uncertainty, with concerns about the duration of response, and the ever-present risk of IRAEs (Watts et al., 2024). Negative impacts on work, finance, hobbies, social life and relationships also feature in patients' experiences (Park et al., 2020; Ala-Leppilami et al., 2020). Cessation of treatment, at the end of the planned course or due to IRAEs, is also a time of difficulty as it heightens concerns about the next steps and the possibility of recurrence (Jamieson et al., 2020). In the future it is anticipated that evidence will emerge on the effectiveness of treatments combining chemotherapy and immunotherapy agents.

Treatment decision-making

Treatment-decision making in advanced cancer can be a difficult and emotionally charged experience (Watts et al., 2024). The context can be particularly challenging for patients with mesothelioma as they are aware they have an incurable cancer with relatively limited treatment options (Bibby et al., 2022).

The relatively small survival benefit associated with chemotherapy may influence some patient's decisions about receiving this treatment. Studies reveal that patients with advanced cancer often decide to go ahead with chemotherapy even when there may be limited benefits to survival (Visser et al., 2018). However, there is also evidence that patients with mesothelioma may weigh up the potential benefits of disease response or stability against the impact on their physical fitness and overall quality of life and decline chemotherapy (Bibby et al., 2022). This decision-making process was captured in an interview study where a wife described her husband's thoughts about chemotherapy *"he looked at it from a much more practical side, went into all the statistics and found out how short a time it would prolong his life and thought well, on balance, it's not worth it"* (Bibby et al., 2022, p. 5)

Immunotherapy presents a new set of challenges for decision-making. Healthcare staff need to find ways to support patients to make treatment decisions in the face of prognostic uncertainty and the inability to predict IRAEs (Watts et al., 2024). Patients view immunotherapy as a source of hope and a chance to extend their lives (Ala-Leppilampi et al., 2020). This creates a difficult context for discussions about treatment which need to manage patient expectations in the light of "exceptional responders" (Wiesenthal et al., 2018) and communicate the uncertainty of the impact of treatment on outcomes (Park et al., 2020). This conversation is likely to be particularly difficult when treatment with immunotherapy is not clinically appropriate, but patients are aware of its potential positive outcomes.

Access to treatment

Inequalities in access to treatment for patients with mesothelioma have been highlighted. Patients describe different approaches depending on the team they have been referred to with some being offered limited treatment options (Johnson et al., 2022). Clinical trials are one way in which patients can access new treatments and referral to centres offering trials are vital to ensuring equity. However, not all patients are referred automatically to centres running mesothelioma clinical trials and some patients have to take their own actions to achieve this (Johnson et al., 2022).

This lack of co-ordination and consistency experienced by some patients suggests a need for regional mesothelioma centres and care systems where patients are automatically referred for specialist review. An example is the Scottish Mesothelioma Network which brings together clinicians across Scotland in order to improve collaboration and promote high-quality, equitable care and access to clinical trials.

There are challenges for patients where standard treatment and care or clinical trials are based in regional centres, unless the resources are in place to overcome them. Patients face the potential burden of long-distance travel with negative financial, time, work and social life implications (Warnock et al., 2019). The split between local and specialist care can also impact on the availability of easily accessible specialist advice and emergency care for the complications of mesothelioma and its treatment. This is particularly important for patients receiving immunotherapy as IRAEs can be difficult to recognise and there may be a lack of knowledge about their management outside of specialist oncology units (Jamieson et al., 2020).

Management options for malignant pleural effusions

Ninety per cent of people with pleural mesothelioma develop a malignant pleural effusion (MPE) at some point in their disease pathway (Bibby et al., 2019). MPE is a condition where fluid builds up around the outside of the lung, between the lung and chest wall. This commonly causes breathlessness and sometimes pain, impacting negatively on QoL. For most people, removal of the fluid improves their symptoms, and there are several methods for achieving this.

One approach to fluid removal is simple therapeutic aspiration, where a plastic cannula is inserted into the fluid (under local anaesthetic) and up to two litres of fluid is aspirated. It is not a long-term solution as the fluid often returns. Despite the short-lived symptom relief, patients consider it to be a worthwhile procedure "*what you go through is worthwhile if you come out as good as I think I have come out*" (Twose et al., 2020).

Recurrence of MPE is common and patients will often require more definitive management. Options include administering an inflammatory agent into the chest cavity to cause the pleural layers to fuse and prevent further fluid build-up. This procedure is called pleurodesis. In the UK and Europe, it involves the use of medical grade talc delivered into the chest either as a slurry via a chest drain or sprayed as a powder (poudrage) during local anaesthetic thoracoscopy. Patients have described the sensation during and post procedure as discomfort rather than pain (Clayson, 2007). The procedure requires an in-patient hospital stay.

An alternative outpatient fluid management strategy is the insertion of an indwelling pleural catheter (IPC). This is a semi-permanent tube that can be inserted as a day case. It is then drained in the patient's home by the community nursing team or family members. Positive patient outcomes have been reported; one study found 87% patients experienced an improvement in quality of life post-IPC insertion (Twose et al., 2020) while a patient in another study noted "*a good drain equals better quality of life*" (Dipper, 2024). IPCs are the best treatment option for trapped or non-expandable lung, or if a previous pleurodesis attempt has failed to keep fluid at bay. IPCs have the additional benefit of allowing talc slurry pleurodesis to be undertaken as an outpatient, which can prevent fluid reaccumulation and enable removal of the catheter in a proportion of patients (Bhatnagar et al., 2018). Potential negative outcomes include the risk of blockage or infection, the inconvenience of repeat drainages and having a medical device in situ as a visible reminder of their disease (Kulendrarajah et al., 2021).

New research is exploring the effectiveness of anticancer drugs being delivered directly into the pleural cavity via IPCs in clinical trials, with the aim of concentrating their effect around the tumour and reducing systemic side effects (Bibby et al., 2021; Danson et al., 2020). This remains experimental work. No intra-pleural drugs are currently licensed for mesothelioma.

Given the different but equally effective approaches to managing MPE, it is vital to provide patients with enough information and support to allow them to make a decision that is right for them. Gaining an understanding of patient priorities and preferences is integral to this. For example, do they prefer an inpatient stay for management or do they prefer management as an outpatient. An online tool has been developed by patients, carers and clinicians that can help people choose their priorities: My Pleural Effusion Journey (Grindell et al., 2020) (https://mypleuraleffusionjourney.com/).

Patients can often feel rushed into making a decision due to their recurrent symptoms. In a recent qualitative study, several people commented that things "*progressed too fast*" and they did not "*have enough time to process*" (Kulendrarajah et al., 2021; Addala et al., 2023). It is important to give people sufficient time to consider the options to enable them to make an informed choice. This must be balanced against the speed of fluid build-up and the desire to avoid repeated, non-definitive interventions. Additionally, if systemic therapy is planned, definitive MPE control should be obtained before treatment begins, as otherwise drugs can accumulate in the pleural fluid and worsen toxicity (Herrstedt et al., 1992). This can add to the sense of time pressure around decision making for MPE.

Experience of malignant pleural effusion management

Patients need close monitoring once diagnosed with MPE to ensure their effusion is managed effectively and minimise the impact it has on their quality of life. There are currently no UK national guidelines for clinicians regarding optimal monitoring for patients with MPE and strategies vary greatly throughout the UK. Managing MPE is complex as every patient is unique with regards to reaccumulation rates, amount of fluid produced, patient reported symptoms and whether patients are receiving anticancer treatment. A recent patient consultation revealed that easy access to a pleural team with regular telephone contact was found to be reassuring to patients and their carers and helped to avoid emergency hospital admissions.

Patients with peritoneal mesothelioma may develop fluid build-up in their abdomen called asities. This can be managed with repeated aspirations or with an indwelling catheter similar to the one for the pleura.

IMPLICATIONS FOR POLICY/PRACTICE

Treatment options for mesothelioma are not curative and provide ways to help managing symptoms, extend life expectancy and optimise quality of life. Decisions about treatment must be patient focused, with a personalised approach to treatment tailored to the individual. Patients and their families and carers require support with decision-making, including advocating for clinical trials and access to new treatments.

Clinical services for mesothelioma treatment pathways should be designed recognising the need for specialist support and advice for a rare cancer with limited treatment options to support care during and post treatment. Specialist nurses play an important role in the delivery and effectiveness of these services.

New treatments with uncertain outcomes and side effects present challenges for providing information to support patients when making treatment decisions. Initiatives such as co-designing information with patients and developing decision support tools should be considered. The uncertainty that accompanies immunotherapy outcomes and IRAEs over a prolonged period may need new and sustained models of care for mesothelioma patients receiving these treatments.

Shortcomings in knowledge among mesothelioma treatments among staff in generalist primary and secondary settings have been identified and need to be addressed.

Early discussions on long term management of MPE are important so patients can consider various MPE management options, and it is important to understand patient priorities to help support the decision process. Having easy access to pleural teams in hospital to encourage patient-initiated follow-up when MPE symptoms occur can help avoid unnecessary hospital admissions.

REFERENCES

Addala, D., Iqbal, B., Denniston, P., et al. (2023). Qualitative study of patient priorities in the malignant pleural effusion pathway. *European Respiratory Journal*, 62(Suppl 67), OA1561. https://doi.org/10.1183/13993003.congress-2023.OA1561

Ala-Leppilampi, K., Baker, N.A., McKillop, C., Butler, M.O., Siu, L.L., Spreafico, A. & Hansen, A.R. (2020). Cancer patients' experiences with immune checkpoint modulators: A qualitative study. *Cancer Medicine*, 9(9), pp. 3015–3022. https://doi.org/10.1002/cam4.2940

Baas, P., et al. (2021). First-line nivolumab plus ipilimumab in unresectable malignant pleural mesothelioma (CheckMate 743): a multicentre, randomised, open-label, phase 3 trial. *The Lancet*, 397(10272), pp. 375–386. https://doi.org/10.1016/S0140-6736(20)32714-8

Bayman, N., et al. (2019). Prophylactic irradiation of tracts in patients with malignant pleural mesothelioma: an open-label, multicenter, phase iii randomized trial. *Journal of Clinical Oncology*, 37(14), pp. 1200–1208. https://doi.org/10.1200/jco.18.01678

Bhatnagar, R., et al. (2018). Outpatient talc administration by indwelling pleural catheter for malignant effusion. *New England Journal of Medicine*, 378(14), 1313–1322.

Bibby, A.C., et al. (2019). The prevalence and clinical relevance of non-expandable lung in malignant pleural mesothelioma: A prospective, single-center cohort study of 229 patients. *Annals of the American Thoracic Society*, 16(10). https://doi.org/10.1513/AnnalsATS.201811-786OC

Bibby, A.C., Morley, A.J., Keenan, E., Maskell, N.A. & Gooberman-Hill, R. (2022). The priorities of people with mesothelioma and their carers: A qualitative interview study of trial participation and treatment decisions. *European Journal of Oncology Nursing*, 57, p. 102111. https://doi.org/10.1016/j.ejon.2022.102111

Bibby, A.C., et al. (2021). A trial of intra-pleural bacterial immunotherapy in malignant pleural mesothelioma (TILT) – A randomised feasibility study using the trial within a cohort (TwiC) methodology. *Europe PMC* (pre-print). https://doi.org/10.21203/rs.3.rs-256386/v2

Clayson H. (2007). *The experience of mesothelioma in Northern England*. PhD thesis, University of Sheffield.

Clive, A.O., et al (2016). Prophylactic radiotherapy for the prevention of procedure-tract metastases after surgical and large-bore pleural procedures in malignant pleural mesothelioma (SMART): a multicentre, open-label, phase 3, randomised controlled trial. *Lancet Oncology*. https://doi.org/10.1016/S1470-2045(16)30095-X

Danson, S.J., et al. (2020). Oncolytic herpesvirus therapy for mesothelioma – A phase I/IIa trial of intrapleural administration of HSV1716. *Lung Cancer*, 150, pp. 145–151. https://doi.org/10.1016/j.lungcan.2020.10.007

Dipper, A. (2024). *Optimising the management of malignant pleural effusion*. PhD thesis, University of Bristol. Available at: https://research-information.bris.ac.uk/en/studentTheses/optimising-the-management-of-malignant-pleural-effusion

Fennell, D.A., et al. (2021). Nivolumab versus placebo in patients with relapsed malignant mesothelioma (CONFIRM): A multicentre, double-blind, randomised, phase 3 trial. *Lancet Oncology*, 22(11), pp. 1530–1540. https://doi.org/10.1016/s1470-2045(21)00471-x

Grindell, C., et al. (2020). Using creative co-design to develop a decision support tool for people with malignant pleural effusion. *Medical Informatics and Decision Making*, 20, p. 179.

Grosso, F., Cerbone, L. & Curioni-Fontecedro, A. (2024). MARS 2 trial: The future of pleurectomy decortication in pleural mesothelioma. *The Lancet Respiratory Medicine*, 12(6), pp. 423–424.

Herrstedt, J., Clementsen, P. & Hansen, O.P. (1992). Increased myelosuppression during cytostatic treatment and pleural effusion in patients with small cell lung cancer. *European Journal of Cancer*, 28a(6–7), pp. 1070–1073. https://doi.org/10.1016/0959-8049(92)90459-f

Jamieson, L., et al. (2020). Immunotherapy and associated immune-related adverse events at a large UK centre: A mixed methods study. *BMC Cancer*, 20(1), p. 743. https://doi.org/10.1186/s12885-020-07215-3

Johnson, M., Allmark, P. & Tod, A. (2022). Living beyond expectations: A qualitative study into the experience of long-term survivors with pleural mesothelioma and their carers. *BMJ Open Respiratory Research*, 9(1), p. e001252. https://doi.org/10.1136/bmjresp-2022-001252

Kulendrarajah, B., George, V. & Rahman, N. (2021). P210 Patient perspectives on pathways in malignant pleural disease: a qualitative study. *Thorax*, 76(Suppl 1), p. A203. https://doi.org/10.1136/thorax-2020-BTSabstracts.355

Lim, E., et al. (2024). Extended pleurectomy decortication and chemotherapy versus chemotherapy alone for pleural mesothelioma (MARS 2): A phase 3 randomised controlled trial. *The Lancet Respiratory Medicine*, 12(6), pp. 457–466.

Lond, B., Apps, L., Quincey, K. & Williamson, I. (2024). The psychological impact of living with peritoneal mesothelioma: An interpretative phenomenological analysis. *Journal of Health Psychology*. https://doi.org/10.1177/13591053241298932

Macleod, N., et al. (2014). Radiotherapy for the treatment of pain in malignant pleural mesothelioma: A systematic review. *Lung Cancer*, 83(2), pp. 133–138. https://doi.org/10.1016/j.lungcan.2013.11.004

Park, R., Shaw, J.W., Korn, A. & McAuliffe, J. (2020). The value of immunotherapy for survivors of stage IV non-small cell lung cancer: Patient perspectives on quality of life. *Journal of Cancer Survivorship*, 14(3), pp. 363–376. https://doi.org/10.1007/s11764-020-00853-3

Rintoul, R.C., et al. (2014). Efficacy and cost of video-assisted thoracoscopic partial pleurectomy versus talc pleurodesis in patients with malignant pleural mesothelioma (MesoVATS): An open-label, randomised, controlled trial. *Lancet*, 384(9948), pp. 1118–11127.

Royal College of Physicians (2020). *National Mesothelioma Audit report 2020 (for the audit period 2016–18)*. London: RCP.

Scherpereel, A., et al. (2020). ERS/ESTS/EACTS/ESTRO guidelines for the management of malignant pleural mesothelioma. *European Respiratory Journal*, 55(6), p. 1900953. https://doi.org/10.1183/13993003.00953-2019

Schmid, S., et al. (2024). Immediate versus deferred systemic therapy in patients with mesothelioma. *Clinical Lung Cancer*, 25(7).

Szlosarek, P.W., et al. (2024). Pegargiminase plus first-line chemotherapy in patients with nonepithelioid pleural mesothelioma: The ATOMIC-Meso randomized clinical trial. *JAMA Oncology*, 10(4), pp. 475–483. https://doi.org/10.1001/jamaoncol.2023.6789

Treasure, T., et al. (2011). Extra-pleural pneumonectomy versus no extra-pleural pneumonectomy for patients with malignant pleural mesothelioma: Clinical outcomes of the Mesothelioma and Radical Surgery (MARS) randomised feasibility study. *Lancet Oncology*, 12(8), pp. 763–772.

Twose, C., et al. (2020). Therapeutic thoracentesis symptoms and activity: A qualitative study. *BMJ Supportive & Palliative Care*. https://doi.org/10.1136/bmjspcare-2020-002584

Visser, S., et al. (2018). Treatment satisfaction of patients with advanced non-small-cell lung cancer receiving platinum-based chemotherapy: Results from a prospective cohort study (PERSONAL). *Clinical Lung Cancer*, 19(4), pp. e503–e516. https://doi.org/10.1016/j.cllc.2018.03.003

Vogelzang, N.J., et al. (2003). Phase III study of pemetrexed in combination with cisplatin versus cisplatin alone in patients with malignant pleural mesotheliom'. *Journal of Clinical Oncology*, 21(14), pp. 2636–2344.

Warnock, C., Lord, K., Taylor, B. & Tod, A. (2019). Patient experiences of participation in a radical thoracic surgical trial: findings from the Mesothelioma and Radical Surgery Trial 2 (MARS 2). *Trials*, 20(1), p. 598. https://doi.org/10.1186/s13063-019-3692-x

Watts, T., Roche, D. & Csontos, J. (2024). Patients' experiences of cancer immunotherapy with immune checkpoint inhibitors: A systematic review and thematic synthesis. *Journal of Clinical Nursing*, 8 April. https://doi.org/10.1111/jocn.17154

Wiesenthal, A.C., Patel, S.P., LeBlanc, T.W., Roeland, E.J. & Kamal A.H. (2018). Top ten tips for palliative care clinicians caring for cancer patients receiving immunotherapies. *Journal of Palliative Medicine*, 21(5), pp. 694–699. https://doi.org/10.1089/jpm.2018.0107

Woolhouse, I., et al. (2018). British Thoracic Society guideline for the investigation and management of malignant pleural mesothelioma. *Thorax*, 73(Suppl 1), pp. i1–i30.

Zalcman, G., et al. (2016). Bevacizumab for newly diagnosed pleural mesothelioma in the Mesothelioma Avastin Cisplatin Pemetrexed Study (MAPS): A randomised, controlled, open-label, phase 3 trial. *Lancet*, 387(10026), pp. 1405–1414. https://doi.org/10.1016/S0140-6736(15)01238-6

Chapter 6

Symptoms and their management

Donna Wakefield, Rachel Smithers and Anna Bibby

OVERVIEW

People with mesothelioma often experience complex physical and psychological symptoms. Previous studies have estimated that approximately 90% of people with pleural mesothelioma present with breathlessness and pain (Moore et al., 2009). The majority experience three or more symptoms, including cough, fatigue, night sweats and low mood (Bibby et al., 2019). For people with peritoneal mesothelioma, abdominal pain and distension are the most common presenting complaints, alongside nausea, vomiting and constipation.

The high symptom burden associated with mesothelioma can negatively impact the quality of life of patients and those supporting them (Moore et al., 2023). Although there is no cure for mesothelioma, treatments to improve survival and symptoms have progressed greatly in the past decade (see Chapters 2 and 5). However, the limited prognosis means that patients and carers must have rapid and easy access to support for their physical, psychological and spiritual needs to optimise their quality of life and future planning.

Current guidelines recognise palliative care as an essential component of symptom control (Woolhouse et al., 2018). Notably, palliative care should not be reserved for the "end-of-life" stage, as patients and carers can benefit from symptomatic and psychological support at any point in their disease trajectory (Brims et al., 2019). Many aspects of this care can be delivered in the community by GPs and nurses or by hospital-based healthcare professionals. Some patients with more complex symptoms may benefit from timely referral to specialist palliative care for more intensive management and support. Specialist palliative care services can provide a holistic approach to patients' needs by focusing on quality of life through optimising symptoms and carer support (Brims et al., 2019). They can also address psychological distress arising from issues related to the industrial nature of the

DOI: 10.4324/9781032631318-6

disease, such as claiming compensation and coroner involvement after death (Harrison et al., 2021). Most patients would prefer to avoid frequent admissions to hospital and be cared for at home, yet admissions in the final few months of life are common (Wakefield et al., 2024), timely Advance Care Planning to discuss a person's wishes is an important aspect of palliative care. Ultimately, given the high symptom burden, people with mesothelioma need a collaborative approach between community, hospital and specialist palliative care services.

This chapter focuses on the most common symptoms experienced by people with mesothelioma and how these symptoms can be managed with non-pharmacological, pharmacological and interventional techniques, referencing the most recent evidence base. It will conclude with a summary of implications for policy and practice.

THE EVIDENCE

Breathlessness

Breathlessness is the most common symptom in pleural mesothelioma, occurring in approximately 70% of patients at presentation and in 80–95% during the disease (Bibby et al., 2019). Breathlessness is frequently reported as the most distressing symptom for patients, significantly impacting daily functioning and quality of life. Management of breathlessness involves an understanding of the impact on daily living and identification of the causes. Some causes of breathlessness can be reversible or improved with interventions. However, breathlessness is often multifactorial and, consequently, requires a multimodal approach to management.

The commonest cause of breathlessness in mesothelioma is a malignant pleural effusion (further details below), which may be drained to improve symptoms (see Chapter 5). However, breathlessness can also occur in the absence of a pleural effusion, usually caused by restriction of respiratory dynamics due to circumferential tumour growth (Bibby et al., 2019). This can be particularly problematic in bulky or advanced disease, where tumours can fully or partially encase the lung, chest wall and/or diaphragm.

Other causes of breathlessness include factors related to mesothelioma and its treatment, such as disease progression, respiratory infection, pulmonary emboli or drug-induced pneumonitis. Extra-thoracic drivers of breathlessness include anaemia, muscle wasting due to deconditioning or steroid treatment, and psychological aspects like anxiety or panic. Exacerbations of pre-existing respiratory conditions, such as chronic obstructive pulmonary disease (COPD) or pulmonary fibrosis, may also contribute to breathlessness.

Pleural interventions

Over 80% of people with pleural mesothelioma develop fluid build-up around the outside of the lung, called a malignant pleural effusion (see Chapter 5) (Bibby et al., 2019). This is a potential reversible cause of breathlessness if the person is well enough to undergo intervention to drain this fluid. Short-term drainage options include therapeutic aspiration or chest drain insertion. Longer-term options involve insertion of an indwelling pleural catheter or talc pleurodesis (Roberts et al., 2023). Chapter 5 provides detailed insight into these methods, including their relative utility, benefits and disadvantages.

Around one-third of people with malignant pleural effusion due to pleural mesothelioma have non-expandable lung (Bibby et al., 2019). This is where the lung cannot inflate due to being surrounded by thickened pleura, leading to breathlessness that may persist despite fluid removal. In these cases, therapeutic aspiration (removing some fluid with a syringe) can provide some symptomatic benefit by reducing pressure on the diaphragm and respiratory muscles (Bibby et al., 2019). Repeated aspiration can be used for people with a short prognosis or where fluid is slow to reaccumulate. If more definitive intervention is required for non-expandable lung, insertion of an indwelling pleural catheter is preferred (Roberts et al., 2023). Aggressive drainage should be avoided, as this can cause chest pain due to negative intrathoracic pressures. Pleurodesis should also be avoided, as it is unlikely to succeed and can result in a complex pleural cavity that is difficult to manage (Roberts et al., 2023). Historically, some patients underwent surgery to release non-expandable lung, however, a recent trial found that this surgery is associated with a shorter prognosis and poorer quality of life in mesothelioma (Lim et al., 2024). Therefore, surgery is performed rarely in the UK.

All procedures necessitate hospital attendance on at least one occasion and are associated with risks and benefits. Therefore, shared decision-making should be used to determine whether this is appropriate and in the patient's best interests.

Non-pharmacological management

Non-pharmacological interventions for breathlessness include using a hand-held fan to deliver airflow across the face. This acts as cheap, portable and highly effective way for patients to self-manage their breathlessness (Gupta et al., 2021). Patients may benefit from learning how specific postures and positions can reduce breathlessness and aid recovery following exertion. Pacing (i.e. deliberately slowing activity speed) and prioritising (i.e. not trying to achieve too much at once) can help people maintain activities of daily living without becoming too breathless (Hui et al., 2020). Other self-management strategies include breathing control exercises to help patients calm their respiratory pattern and avoid anxiety exacerbating their symptoms (Wood et al., 2012). Palliative oxygen is not recommended unless patients are hypoxic, with oxygen saturations <90% (Abernethy et al., 2010).

Clinicians must recognise and explicitly acknowledge to patients that breathlessness is very frightening. Indeed, many report feeling as if they are "about to die", which can understandably trigger panic and anxiety and, in turn, worsen symptoms. Alongside breathing control exercises, Cognitive Behavioural Therapy (CBT) may reduce panic and breathlessness for some patients (Hui et al., 2020).

Pharmacological management

Most people with breathlessness due to cancer will require pharmacological treatment in addition to non-pharmacological strategies. Opioids have been used for many years to manage breathlessness. They work in various ways, including reducing the central response to hypercapnia, hypoxia and exertion, to reduce respiratory efforts. Opioids also appear to modify people's perception of breathlessness and anticipatory breathlessness.

The strongest evidence for opioids to relieve breathlessness is for regular low-dose oral morphine, e.g. 5mg twice daily (Johnson & Currow, 2020). Whilst modified release preparations provide more consistent relief, with fewer fluctuations in opioid plasma concentrations, anecdotally, some people benefit from immediate release morphine (e.g. oramorph), particularly when taken pre-emptively before exertion (Hui et al., 2020). Low doses are usually effective for breathlessness and, in contrast to pain management, the maximum effective dose is around 30mg of modified release morphine in 24 hours. Importantly, not all patients will benefit from an opioid and further titration risks undesirable side effects, including the risk of respiratory depression (Johnson & Currow, 2020).

There is a lack of evidence to support the routine use of benzodiazepines (such as lorazepam or diazepam). However, they can be effective to relieve breathlessness for those where there is a strong anxiety/panic response related to breathlessness (Hui et al., 2020).

People with low oxygen levels on exertion or at rest may benefit from palliative or ambulatory oxygen (Abernethy et al., 2010). Unlike long-term oxygen therapy for people with COPD, oxygen does not confer any survival benefit.

Pain

Chest pain is present in approximately 60% of people presenting with pleural mesothelioma, and it appears to be more common in people without pleural effusions (Bibby et al., 2019). Pain severity varies over the disease course and may escalate in the pre-terminal phase. Mild pain is relatively common, while moderate or severe pain (graded as a score more than 40 on a 100mm visual analogue scale) was only reported in 21 of 140 (14%) people in a recent UK multicentre observational study (Mayland et al., 2024). Nonetheless, where moderate or severe pain was present, it impacted on people's quality of life and interfered with their daily activities. In pleural mesothelioma, the presence of pain at diagnosis has been associated with shorter survival, potentially as it indicates more aggressive or advanced disease (Bibby et al., 2019).

In peritoneal mesothelioma, abdominal pain is common, arising from abdominal distention due to a build-up of ascitic fluid or tumour invasion of abdominal structures. Disruption of bowel function secondary to tumour obstruction or nerve involvement can also cause abdominal discomfort. Depending on the underlying cause, large volume ascitic drainage, indwelling abdominal catheter insertion or laxatives can be helpful, alongside the World Health Organisation's (WHO) analgesic ladder approach.

Pharmacological management

Systemic analgesia is the first-line treatment for pain, with the WHO analgesic ladder for cancer pain being the cornerstone of pharmacological management (Ventafridda et al., 1985). This stepwise approach recommends starting with simple analgesia, such as nonsteroidal anti-inflammatory drugs and paracetamol, followed by weak then strong opioids, such as morphine, if required. Although for moderate-severe cancer pain it is common practice to directly start at WHO analgesic ladder step 3, by initiating a low-dose strong opioid.

When considering medication routes, the WHO recommends oral medication wherever possible to allow patients greater control and independence in managing their pain (Ventafridda et al., 1985). Additionally, the WHO suggests giving modified or slow-release analgesia at regular intervals, with faster-acting medication used for breakthrough pain. Adjuvant analgesics can be added at any step in the analgesic ladder, for example, for patients with neuropathic elements to their pain.

Neuropathic pain is relatively common in pleural mesothelioma due to the proximity of the pleura and therefore the tumour to the thoracic neurovascular bundle that carries the intercostal nerves. Neuropathic agents, such as gabapentin, pregabalin or amitriptyline may be useful adjuncts to opioid analgesia if neuropathic pain is present.

Interventions

Interventional therapies can be used for severe or non-opioid responsive mesothelioma pain. For instance, peripheral nerve blocks involve injection of local anaesthetic or ablative agents to reduce or block nerve-related pain signals (Saunders et al., 2019). These are effective when a single nerve or nerve root is affected.

Palliative radiotherapy can provide pain reduction across a wider area than nerve blocks. However, pain must align with areas of radiologically demonstrated disease to enable radiotherapy planning and targeting (Woolhouse et al., 2018). Radiotherapy is also an effective treatment for procedure tract metastases where tumour cells spread along the route of prior interventions, giving rise to painful subcutaneous deposits (Woolhouse et al., 2018). Prophylactic irradiation is not required, as subsequent metastases often respond rapidly to directed radiotherapy (Woolhouse et al., 2018).

A small number of people with pleural mesothelioma experience severe chest pain that persists despite maximal pharmacological treatment. This often requires more invasive management through percutaneous cervical cordotomy (PCC). PCC utilises radiofrequency ablation to interrupt nerves in the spinal cord, thereby preventing pain signals from reaching the brain. Consequently, PCC is very effective for localised unilateral pain, with one meta-analysis of 160 patients undergoing PCC showing good pain relief in the majority, with some patients able to stop opioid medication completely (France et al., 2013). However, some degree of pain returned for 34% of patients post-PCC, with a greater incidence as time passed. Despite this, the overall effectiveness of PCC means that the National Mesothelioma Framework recommends it as an adjuvant to analgesia at any stage in the WHO ladder. Unfortunately, in the UK, access to PCC is hindered by limited provision and geographical barriers, with only four NHS centres currently offering it.

Cough

While cough is less common in pleural mesothelioma, it still affects around 40% of people at diagnosis and is more common in those with pleural effusions, and non-expandable lung (Bibby et al., 2019). Cough can be distressing and embarrassing for patients and can cause or exacerbate chest pain and breathlessness. Unfortunately, cough is challenging to treat.

Non-pharmacological management

Non-pharmacological measures include regular sips of fluid, cough sweets or lozenges and soothing drinks like hot honey and lemon. Clinicians should treat common non-mesothelioma causes, e.g. gastro-oesophageal reflux or upper airway disease, and be aware of other respiratory pathologies that may co-exist, e.g. COPD or asbestos-related pulmonary fibrosis.

Pharmacological management

Where cough persists despite optimising alternate causes or is thought to be cancer-related, cough suppressants of increasing strength can be used, following a stepwise approach. UK guidelines suggest that simple linctus should be trialled initially, followed by a weak opioid, such as codeine or pholcodine linctus, and, finally, a low-dose strong opioid like oral morphine (NICE, 2023). While neuropathic agents, including gabapentin and pregabalin, are effective cough suppressants, side effects limit their common use. Newer drugs that block afferent nerve messaging and disrupt the cough hypersensitivity reflex are currently under investigation in clinical trials.

Cough in pleural mesothelioma does not seem to respond to anticancer treatment. Indeed, radiotherapy may transiently worsen cough, and immunotherapy can cause drug-induced pneumonitis and cough. In people with pleural effusion, over-drainage can worsen symptoms, especially in those with non-expandable lung.

Systemic symptoms

Systemic symptoms such as lethargy, low appetite and weight loss are present in at least 20% of people with mesothelioma and often become more prominent as the disease progresses (Bibby et al., 2019). Hot flushes, fevers and sweats also affect mesothelioma patients and can be distressing and uncomfortable. These symptoms reflect increased levels of pro-inflammatory cytokines, such as tumour necrosis factor, interleukin-6 and interferon-gamma, released by activated immune cells in response to tumour antigens.

Non-pharmacological management

A hand-held fan or cold flannel can help ease hot flushes or sweating, while advice to eat "little and often" may enhance oral intake in the context of poor appetite. Nutritional supplements, including build-up drinks, can prevent dramatic weight loss, but many people find them unpalatable. For cancer-related fatigue, if able, light aerobic exercise, yoga and/or CBT can help. Whilst there is no evidence that any medications have a clinical impact (including a recent trial which confirmed methylphenidate was of no benefit (Stone et al., 2024)).

Pharmacological management

Simple anti-inflammatory medication like NSAIDs may provide some relief and should be trialled first. Oral corticosteroids can improve systemic symptoms by inhibiting inflammatory cascades, whilst also stimulating appetite and weight gain (Arends et al., 2021). However, the palliative effects of corticosteroids are often transient, and in the longer term, their adverse effects, particularly loss of muscle mass and limb strength, can negatively impact patients' functional ability and quality of life. Consequently, the European Society for Medical Oncology recommends corticosteroids for 2–3 weeks, repeated periodically if patients find them beneficial (Arends et al., 2021).

The synthetic progestogen megestrol acetate has been shown to improve appetite and quality of life in people with cancer and support minor weight gain (Arends et al., 2021). However, side effects, including thromboembolic events, can increase morbidity and mortality in patients treated with megestrol so people must be counselled about potential risks to allow an informed decision about whether they wish to try it.

Gastrointestinal symptoms

Nausea, vomiting and constipation can occur in people with mesothelioma either due to peritoneal disease or treatment side effects. Chemotherapy is renowned for causing significant nausea and vomiting, while one of the most serious potential side effects of immunotherapy is diarrhoea due to colitis. Opioids commonly cause constipation, as can some anti-sickness (antiemetic) medications like ondansetron. If severe, constipation can worsen nausea.

Malignant bowel obstruction must be considered in people with peritoneal mesothelioma who have sudden-onset nausea and vomiting with worsening abdominal pain or distension.

Pharmacological management

Laxatives and antiemetics are the mainstay of treatment for constipation and nausea respectively. Both medications should be prescribed prophylactically for all patients using regular opioids (Hui et al., 2020), although there is a lack of direct evidence to guide drug selection. Clinicians may recommend a specific antiemetic based on suspected underlying cause or mechanism. For example, nausea arising from other drugs, such as morphine, may respond best to antiemetics that work on the chemoreceptor trigger zone, e.g. haloperidol. Other factors to consider when choosing an antiemetic include availability, side effects, route and patient preference. There is similarly limited evidence for the superiority of any particular laxative, with drug selection based on expert opinion and guided by the patient's history and preference. For prophylaxis of opioid-induced constipation, a stimulant laxative like senna is often the first choice.

Malignant bowel obstruction may require surgical or endoscopic interventions. However, if constipation or volvulus (twisting of the bowel) is the cause, conservative management with laxatives and a flatus tube may be effective. Sadly, in many cases, bowel obstruction represents a terminal event. Therefore, palliation and end-of-life planning may be the best course of treatment (see Chapter 9). This should include antisecretory and antiemetic drugs to ameliorate nausea, vomiting and pain. Vomiting related to bowel obstruction may be relieved by inserting a nasogastric tube. However, this is an uncomfortable procedure, and people may not like having the tube in place, so its use should be weighed against the severity of the vomiting and patient preference.

Psychological symptoms

Mesothelioma is a devastating diagnosis. Its incurable nature, limited life expectancy and high symptom burden can lead to feelings of hopelessness and anxiety about the future. Uncertainty regarding prognosis and treatment can compound these feelings (Bibby et al., 2022). The occupational element of mesothelioma and asbestos exposure can generate complex feelings of anger and blame, as well as anxiety about colleagues/friends who may be affected (Guglielmucci et al., 2018). These disease-specific factors mean that depression and anxiety are reported frequently by people with mesothelioma and their family members (Harrison et al., 2021). Chapter 12 covers mental health and wellbeing in greater detail, including potential strategies to overcome negative psychological symptoms. Generally, managing psychological symptoms in people with mesothelioma reflects modalities used in the general population, namely combining psychotherapeutic and pharmacological measures.

Non-pharmacological management

The British Thoracic Society (BTS), European Respiratory Society and Mesothelioma UK all stress the importance of palliative care in ensuring holistic assessment and management of people's psychological, emotional and spiritual needs. According to the BTS guidelines, all people with mesothelioma must have a named, contactable key worker within the multidisciplinary team managing their care (Woolhouse et al., 2018). These key workers are often mesothelioma specialist nurses who can offer invaluable practical and emotional support and provide continuity of care throughout people's disease journey and the different services and treatments they access. However, some people may require more expert support, including formal psychotherapeutic strategies, such as CBT and psychoeducation for anxiety symptoms.

The primary source of support for patients with mesothelioma is often their family and friends. It is evident from qualitative studies that adopting a caring role, as frequently necessitated by the disease, has a significant impact on the physical, emotional and social wellbeing of caregivers (see Chapters 10 and 12). Palliative care specialists are essential to addressing carers' unmet needs (see Chapter 9). By viewing patients as the centre of wider support networks, palliative care specialists seek to assess and manage carer needs as an integral part of patient care (Harrison et al., 2021).

Pharmacological management

Antidepressants are recommended based on the observed benefits in the general population. Selective serotonin reuptake inhibitors like sertraline are often started first due to better tolerability and fewer side effects. Alternative class antidepressants may be preferred in some cases, like mirtazapine, where insomnia and poor appetite are problematic. Potential side effects should always be considered.

IMPLICATIONS FOR POLICY/PRACTICE

Mesothelioma presents unique challenges in symptom management due to its high symptom burden and unique disease characteristics. Recognising the multidimensional nature of symptoms allows a multimodal management approach that optimises effective symptom control. Clinicians should seek to combine non-pharmacological, pharmacological and interventional strategies to ensure patients are as symptom-free as possible.

Specialist palliative care may not be necessary for everyone, although it is indicated for complex or intractable symptoms. Services aim to optimise physical, emotional, psychological, spiritual and social wellbeing to enhance wellbeing and achieve maximal quality of life. This aim must be communicated to patients and their families before referral to address the misconception that palliative care is synonymous with end-of-life care.

Percutaneous cervical cordotomy is a very effective intervention for relieving intractable, unilateral pain, especially with a neuropathic element. The limited number of centres in the UK providing this service is problematic as it precludes access for some patients, particularly for those who are significantly debilitated. Professionals treating people with mesothelioma must be aware of their nearest centre and be able to support access to the procedure. Charitable organisations like Mesothelioma UK can provide practical and financial support to access PCC services.

The impact of physical symptoms can result in psychological and emotional distress that, in turn, exacerbates symptoms, causing a "vicious circle". According to the Mesothelioma Service Framework, all patients should have a named and contactable key worker within the multidisciplinary team. This is often a mesothelioma specialist nurse, hence, ideally all hospitals caring for people with mesothelioma should have access to this resource.

Ultimately, management of mesothelioma symptoms demands a holistic approach supported by the multidisciplinary team and cross-sector agencies in hospitals and the community. By addressing all elements of the symptom burden associated with mesothelioma, people with mesothelioma and their caregivers' wellbeing can be optimised, resulting in the best quality of life, regardless of prognosis.

REFERENCES

Abernethy, A.P., et al. (2010). Effect of palliative oxygen versus room air in relief of breathlessness in patients with refractory dyspnoea: A double-blind, randomised controlled trial. *The Lancet*, 376(9743), pp. 784–793.

Arends, J., et al. (2021). Cancer cachexia in adult patients: ESMO Clinical Practice Guidelines. *ESMO Open*.

Bibby, A.C., Halford, P., Duneesha De Fonseka, Morley, A.J., Smith, S. & Maskell, N.A. (2019). The prevalence and clinical relevance of nonexpandable lung in malignant pleural mesothelioma. A prospective, single-center cohort study of 229 patients. *Annals of the American Thoracic Society*, 16(10), pp. 1273–1279.

Bibby, A.C., Morley, A.J., Keenan, E., Maskell, N.A. & Gooberman-Hill, R. (2022). The priorities of people with mesothelioma and their carers: A qualitative interview study of trial participation and treatment decisions. *European Journal of Oncology Nursing*, 57, p. 102111.

Brims, F., et al. (2019). Early specialist palliative care on quality of life for malignant pleural mesothelioma: a randomised controlled trial. *Thorax*, 74(4), pp. 354–336.

France, B.D., Lewis, R.A., Sharma, M.L. & Poolman, M. (2013). Cordotomy in mesothelioma-related pain: A systematic review. *BMJ Supportive & Palliative Care*, 4(1), pp. 19–29.

Guglielmucci, F., Franzoi, I.G., Bonafede, M., Borgogno, F.V., Grosso, F. & Granieri, A. (2018). "The less I think about it, the better I feel": A thematic analysis of the subjective experience of malignant mesothelioma patients and their caregivers. *Frontiers in Psychology*, 9.

Gupta, A., et al. (2021). Nonpharmacological interventions for managing breathlessness in patients with advanced cancer. *JAMA Oncology*, 7(2), p. 290.

Harrison, M., Gardiner, C., Taylor, B., Ejegi-Memeh, S. & Darlison, L. (2021). Understanding the palliative care needs and experiences of people with mesothelioma and their family carers: An integrative systematic review. *Palliative Medicine*, 35(6), pp. 1039–1051.

Hui, D., Maddocks, M., Johnson, M.J., Ekström, M., Simon, S.T., Ogliari, A.C., Booth, S. & Ripamonti, C. (2020). Management of breathlessness in patients with cancer: ESMO Clinical Practice Guidelines. *ESMO Open*, 5(6), p. e001038.

Johnson, M.J. & Currow, D.C. (2020). Opioids for breathlessness: A narrative review. *BMJ Supportive & Palliative Care*, 10(3), pp. 287–295.

Lim, E., et al. (2024). Extended pleurectomy decortication and chemotherapy versus chemotherapy alone for pleural mesothelioma (MARS 2): A phase 3 randomised controlled trial. *The Lancet Respiratory Medicine*.

Mayland, C.R., et al. (2024). Unravelling pain in Malignant Pleural Mesothelioma: A longitudinal study [poster]. British Thoracic Society Winter Meeting. November 2024, London.

Moore, A., Bennett, B., Taylor-Stokes, G. & Daumont, M.J. (2023). Caregivers of patients with malignant pleural mesothelioma: Who provides care, what care do they provide and what burden do they experience? *Quality of Life Research*.

Moore, S., Darlinson, L. & Tod, A.M. (2009). Living with mesothelioma. A literature review. *European Journal of Cancer Care*, 19(4), pp. 458–468.

NICE (2023). *Cough.* Available at: https://cks.nice.org.uk/topics/cough/

Roberts, M.E., et al. (2023). British Thoracic Society guideline for pleural disease. *Thorax*, 78(Suppl 3), pp. s1–s42.

Saunders, J., Ashton, M., Hall, C., Laird, B. & MacLeod, N. (2019). Pain management in patients with malignant mesothelioma: Challenges and solutions. *Lung Cancer: Targets and Therapy*, 10, pp. 37–46.

Stone, P.C., Minton, O., Richardson, A., Buckle, P., Enayat, Z.E., Marston, L. & Freemantle, N. (2024). Methylphenidate versus placebo for treating fatigue in patients with advanced cancer: Randomized, double-blind, multicenter, placebo-controlled trial. *Journal of Clinical Oncology*, 42(20), pp. 2382–2392.

Ventafridda, V., Saita, L., Ripamonti, C. & De Conno, F. (1985). WHO guidelines for the use of analgesics in cancer pain. *International Journal of Tissue Reactions*, 7(1), pp. 93–96.

Wakefield, D., Ward, T., Edge, H., Mayland, C.R. & Gardiner C. (2024). Palliative and end-of-life care for patients with pleural mesothelioma: A cohort study. *Palliative Medicine*, 0(0). https://doi.org/10.1177/02692163241302454

Wood, H., Connors, S., Dogan, S. & Peel, T. (2012). Individual experiences and impacts of a physiotherapist-led, non-pharmacological breathlessness programme for patients with intrathoracic malignancy: A qualitative study. *Palliative Medicine*, 27(6), pp. 499–507.

Woolhouse, I., et al. (2018). British Thoracic Society guideline for the investigation and management of malignant pleural mesothelioma. *Thorax*, 73(Suppl 1), pp. i1–i30.

Chapter 7

The supportive care needs of people with mesothelioma

Zoe Davey and Catherine Henshall

OVERVIEW

Mesothelioma is a life-limiting cancer, and most patients enter the best supportive care phase of their cancer pathway soon after diagnosis. Routine follow-up and surveillance are a vital part of the supportive cancer care pathway. Surveillance for mesothelioma patients involves regular monitoring and check-up appointments for the purposes of symptom management and monitoring to see if disease has progressed or remained stable. Follow-up care also involves the holistic provision of psychosocial, emotional, physical, informational and financial support. The care needs of mesothelioma patients can differ to patients with other advanced cancers, requiring expert clinical input and sensitive, managed care that is disease specific. Despite this, there are often substantial regional variations in patients' access to specialist care, as well as differences in clinical decision-making pathways and mesothelioma service structures across healthcare trusts. This chapter will examine the challenges for mesothelioma patients as they navigate the best supportive care pathway and will consider evidence on patients' and family members' experiences of this trajectory. With regards to follow-up care, different models are examined, including the roles of health and social care professionals and services in the delivery of specialist mesothelioma care. Suggestions for how health services can resource and manage mesothelioma follow-up care to provide optimal support for patients and their families during this crucial period of their cancer journey are provided.

DOI: 10.4324/9781032631318-7

THE EVIDENCE

What is follow-up care?

Despite advances in the management of mesothelioma, it is an incurable cancer and treatment options for mesothelioma patients remain limited. The treatments that are available (e.g. immunotherapy, chemotherapy, radiotherapy) are primarily aimed at helping to control symptoms and slow disease progression. Routine follow-up and surveillance are a vital part of the supportive cancer care pathway. They usually begin once a patient has completed their initial first-line treatment, when they may enter a period of follow-up and surveillance between treatments. Other times follow-up and surveillance may begin when the disease has progressed and treatment is stopped. Surveillance for mesothelioma patients involves regular monitoring for signs of disease progression and symptom management; this includes out-patient appointments and imaging scans. For some patients the stage of their disease may be too advanced for treatment aimed at prolonging life to be beneficial, but there are other supportive care treatments that can be used to relieve symptoms, make patients more comfortable and improve quality of life. The provision of supportive cancer care (sometimes referred to as palliative care), encompassing both follow-up and surveillance needs, is specifically concerned with holistic needs assessments and the prevention and management of any psychosocial and physical symptoms of disease, as well as any side effects of cancer and its treatment (for more on palliative care in mesothelioma see Chapter 9). It is also focused on the provision of informational, social and financial support. Throughout this chapter we will refer to supportive care as an umbrella term for both follow-up care and surveillance. Research examining patients' and healthcare professionals' views of cancer follow-up care and surveillance has found that well-organised and regular follow-up care is valued by patients, who find it reassuring to have consistent contact with specialist healthcare professionals (Lewis et al., 2009).

Although best supportive care is routinely provided to all patients with a cancer diagnosis, the follow-up care needs of mesothelioma patients differ to those of other cancer patients, requiring disease-specific clinical input and sensitively managed care (Henshall et al., 2021). For example, in addition to symptom management support, patients and family carers require support in addressing the complex psychosocial and emotional challenges associated with a terminal diagnosis. For patients whose disease is progressing quickly there is limited time to capture deterioration, concerns and issues, and to address them. Moreover, mesothelioma patients and their families often require specific information and guidance on financial and social support issues, including compensation, benefits and coroner requirements.

Currently, there are few long-term survivors of mesothelioma, with most patients living less than 12 months post-diagnosis. However, patients that do survive for longer have specific follow-up and supportive care needs, including managing their expectations of a longer than expected prognosis and navigating longer term surveillance pathways (Johnson et al., 2022).

Published guidance for the diagnosis and treatment of mesothelioma recommends that a personalised approach to follow-up care is considered for each patient, to help determine the frequency of follow-up appointments and scans, and to allow flexibility concerning the need to attend face-to-face clinics or receive regular telephone follow-up, in line with treatment plans and individual patient preferences (Kusamura et al., 2021; Woolhouse et al., 2018).

Who delivers follow-up care?

Within cancer care pathways, approaches to follow-up care can vary depending on where services are based, the frequency of appointments, how care is structured and delivered, and the healthcare professionals involved in providing care. These different models of care can include hospital-based follow-up within specialist cancer centres, nurse-led follow-up and primary care follow-up linked to GP services. Regular follow-up appointments can take place face-to-face, over the phone or be organised ad hoc as part of patient-initiated follow-up. Mesothelioma follow-up care is typically delivered by an oncologist, respiratory physician and/or cancer specialist nurse, depending on the type and stage of cancer and patients' individual treatment plans. Patients under the care of palliative care services or hospice care may also receive follow-up care in community and other out of hospital settings.

It is recommended that follow-up care is delivered by specialist mesothelioma teams to improve management and outcomes (Ball et al., 2016; de Boer et al., 2019). For mesothelioma patients in the United Kingdom, these teams may be led by mesothelioma specialist nurses. There are approximately 31 mesothelioma specialist nurses spread geographically across England and Scotland, currently funded by Mesothelioma UK, who provide care for patients with mesothelioma within the National Health Service (NHS) (Mesothelioma UK, 2024). See Chapter 3 for more information on the role of mesothelioma specialist nurses. Following recommendations from the British Thoracic Society, several specialist mesothelioma multidisciplinary teams (MDTs) have been established to provide expert input into clinical decision-making around the personalised treatment and follow-up of mesothelioma patients (Woolhouse et al., 2018). Despite this, patients with mesothelioma often enter more general follow-up care pathways alongside other lung cancer patients, with specialist services for mesothelioma often only provided within larger tertiary or specialist centres. Patients based in regional and other non-specialist centres are not always able to access these specialist services, leading to disjointed and inequitable care provision (Ball et al., 2016).

What are patient and family members experiences of follow-up care?

There is often substantial geographical variation in patients' ability to access specialist care services, as well as differences in clinical decision-making and the structure of mesothelioma services across healthcare trusts (Henshall et al., 2021; 2022). Patient and family members' experiences of follow-up care are similarly variable. Mesothelioma is a cancer associated with a substantial symptom burden, including fatigue, pain, weight loss, anxiety and low mood, as well as high levels of unmet need (Ejegi-Memeh, 2022; Hoon et al., 2021). Patients and their family members must navigate the healthcare, benefits and legal systems, making difficult decisions around treatment and care, learning how to access benefits and compensation, and adjusting to what it means to receive a mesothelioma diagnosis (Sherborne et al., 2020). In addition, routine surveillance procedures such as scans and clinic assessments can be associated with considerable anxiety (sometimes referred to as 'scanxiety') as patients and their families often encounter delays as they wait for outcomes of procedures to monitor the progression of their disease (Sherborne et al., 2020). The research literature indicates that the experiences and care needs of patients and family members may differ as they move from the point of diagnosis and treatment through to follow-up and end-of-life care (Ejegi-Memeh, 2022).

Whilst there are few long-term survivors of mesothelioma, follow-up care and surveillance can be particularly challenging for patients and family members in this group. Research examining the experiences of long-term survivors with pleural mesothelioma has found that patients have mixed feelings about exceeding survival estimates given at the point of diagnosis. Patients describe the complexities of managing the expectations of families and friends, making longer term life decisions (financial, social, practical), developing effective coping strategies, managing longer term surveillance, adjusting to changes in disease progression and dealing with the symptom burden of prolonged treatment (Johnson et al., 2022).

There is limited research that directly examines experiences of follow-up care for people with mesothelioma, particularly for people diagnosed with peritoneal mesothelioma. Research looking at patients' and family members' experiences of care from the point of diagnosis emphasises the importance of continuity, communication and coordination as crucial influences on positive experiences of care and coping (Ejegi-Memeh, 2022). Research examining malignant pleural mesothelioma patients' and family members' experiences of follow-up care and surveillance has found that despite variations in care, overall perceptions of care tend to be positive, but these perceptions are influenced by four key factors: people, process, place and purpose (Henshall et al., 2021) (see Box 7.1).

BOX 7.1   THE VIEWS OF PEOPLE WITH MESOTHELIOMA ON FACTORS INFLUENCING THEIR EXPERIENCES OF FOLLOW-UP CARE HIGHLIGHTED BY HENSHALL AND COLLEAGUES (2021)

People

Open communication and continuity of care from a named healthcare professional is highly valued. Seeing the same lead consultant or specialist nurse at each follow-up appointment and having sufficient time within each appointment to discuss their condition, is crucial for building confidence in the care pathway. People with mesothelioma often move between different healthcare teams from the point of diagnosis through to treatment and follow-up, and without a consistent point of contact and clear communication, care pathways can become fragmented and difficult to navigate. People with mesothelioma do not always know who they should contact if they require advice in managing their symptoms, dealing with changes in their condition, making decisions around treatment, or accessing other services or forms of support (e.g. financial, social, psychological). In addition to their clinical care teams, the important role of family, friends, and support groups during the follow-up care and surveillance period is pivotal.

Processes and places

When routine systems and processes fail are error-prone, or delayed, significant distress and anxiety can ensue. Examples include delays and difficulty booking appointments, telephone helplines, accessing different services, and receiving and waiting for scan and test results. Similarly, frustrations relate to inefficient, impractical, and difficult to access clinic appointments and hospital sites. People with mesothelioma appreciate when these processes can flex according to their circumstances, as well as being able to meet their individual care needs; this makes navigating follow-up care and surveillance pathways simpler.

Purpose

The importance of regular follow-up consultations with clinical care teams to receive condition specific information to guide decision making, monitor disease progression and manage symptoms is imperative. People with mesothelioma benefit from information and guidance about routes into clinical trials, standard and novel treatment options, benefits and entitlements, and transitions to community and palliative care services. The provision of up-to-date information requires specialist knowledge within clinical care teams and needs to be supported by appropriate resources and information packs. General health literacy and specific knowledge of mesothelioma varies substantially, and information needs to be tailored and delivered at the right time and in the right place. However, people with mesothelioma prioritise good communication more highly than resources alone, emphasising the importance of continuity of care and trusting relationships with members of the clinical team.

Experiences of long-term mesothelioma survivors further highlight the importance of regular input from specialist healthcare professionals, disease-specific and asbestos disease charities, and family carers in meeting supportive care needs over prolonged periods of time (Johnson et al., 2022). There is a need for regular follow-up to monitor disease progression, improve access to psychosocial support and to aid coordination between primary, secondary, palliative and community care services (Johnson et al., 2022).

How should follow-up care be delivered?

Whilst follow-up care and surveillance can differ in terms of which services are involved and when and where care is delivered, research examining patient and family members' experiences of care consistently highlights the key role of the mesothelioma cancer specialist nurse in improving continuity, coordination and confidence in care pathways (Ejegi-Memeh, 2022; Gardiner et al., 2022; Henshall et al., 2021).

Specialist nurses are part of clinical care teams for many different health conditions and can positively impact on patient outcomes and system processes, enhancing continuity and quality of care, and service efficiency (Kerr et al., 2021). They are central to effectively meeting the supportive care needs of people with advanced cancers, including through the provision of specialist and early palliative care, and have been shown to improve patient satisfaction. Specialist nurses can develop meaningful relationships with people with mesothelioma and their families, providing physical, emotional, practical, informational, financial and social support. They also oversee care coordination and communication pathways, facilitate support groups and promote clinical trials opportunities. In addition, specialist nurses are highly valued members of the multidisciplinary team and are central to clinical decision-making and ongoing care planning for people with mesothelioma (Henshall et al., 2022).

Based on the follow-up care preferences of people with pleural mesothelioma, a "Pyramid of Care" model has been conceptualised to outline the requirements for sustainable and patient-centred care pathways (Davey & Henshall, 2021). This approach acknowledges the central role of the specialist nurse, placing them at the top of the pyramid, supported by a named consultant, clinical care team and supportive care services (see Figure 7.1). In addition, recommendations for follow-up

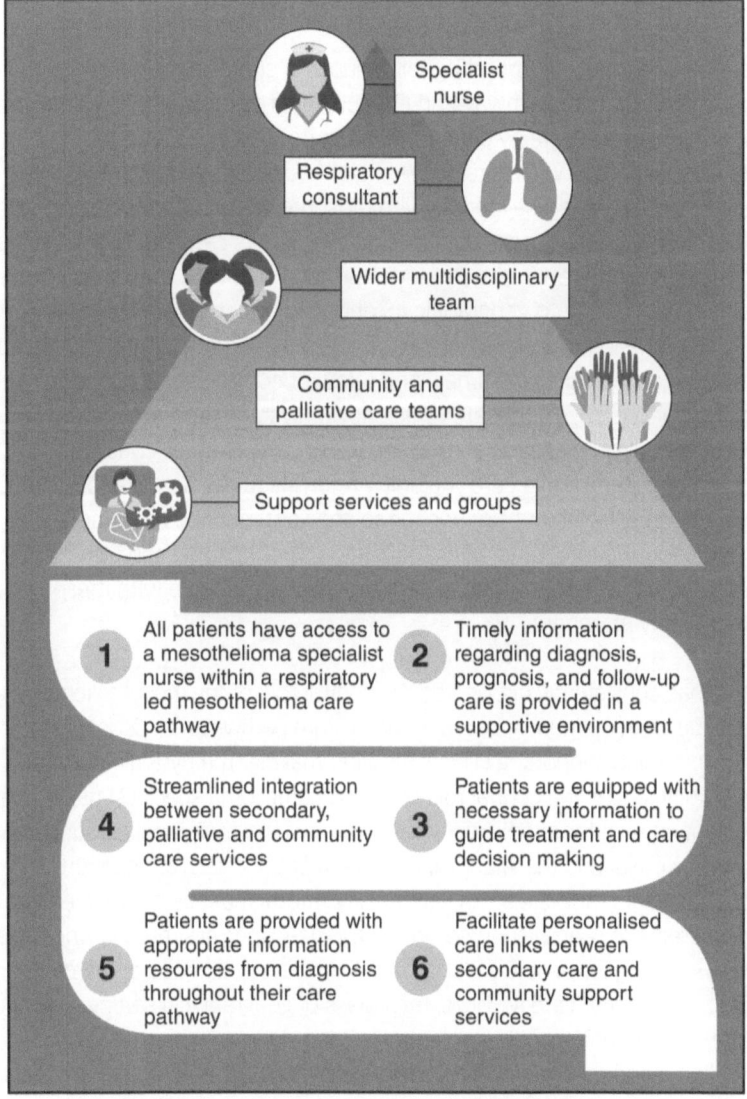

Figure 7.1 Pyramid of Care and recommendations for mesothelioma follow-up care

care developed in conjunction with people with lived experience and healthcare professionals call for specialist nurses to act as the primary point of contact, facilitating continuity of care and reciprocal communication and feedback channels across different services. Specialist nurses can also ensure that relevant, timely specialist information and best supportive care is provided to people with mesothelioma through active involvement in their follow-up and surveillance pathways.

IMPLICATIONS FOR POLICY/PRACTICE

Best supportive care, incorporating follow-up and surveillance, is a vital part of the mesothelioma care pathway and impacts most people with mesothelioma and their families. Despite evidence that most people with mesothelioma require specialist follow-up care delivered by healthcare professionals with condition-specific expertise, people with mesothelioma and their families are often not able to access these specialist services. This can lead to individuals experiencing considerable unmet needs and receiving care that is disjointed and variable according to geographic location and inconsistencies in service set-up and provision. Continuity of care and contact with a named healthcare professional, as well as clear, timely and relevant communication and information provision, and greater efficiency of systems and processes, can all positively impact on individuals' experiences of care. Greater consistency in the delivery of best supportive care, including referrals to regional mesothelioma specialist nurses, improved signposting to specialist services and more joined-up coordination between hospital and out of hospital services can all enhance and contribute to optimal care provision for people with mesothelioma and their family members.

Research has consistently highlighted the central role of the mesothelioma specialist nurse in optimising best supportive care pathways for people with mesothelioma and supporting clinical decision-making. The Pyramid of Care model acknowledges the central role of the mesothelioma specialist nurse as a key point of contact for people with mesothelioma and their families, supported by a named consultant, the wider clinical care team and relevant supportive care services. To ensure consistency in care quality, efforts must be made to ensure that mesothelioma specialist nurses, or lung cancer specialist nurses who have expertise in caring for people with mesothelioma, are positioned at the centre of mesothelioma cancer care services, regardless of geographical setting or service structure. This will enhance their role profiles and will mean that people with mesothelioma and their family members will be more aware of how the specialist nurses can optimise their experiences of care from the start of their cancer care pathway onwards.

It is also key that people with mesothelioma are provided with a named point of contact to help coordinate and navigate the complex, variable and often unpredictable nature of their care pathways. Identifying a specialist nurse at the outset and providing a clear explanation of how they can be reached and the extent of the support they are able to provide may increase the confidence of people with mesothelioma and their families to seek support when it is needed, rather than waiting until their care and support needs have escalated. This may result in more individuals receiving care and support for their holistic care needs at an earlier stage, reducing the potential for difficulties in the management of their care.

People with mesothelioma frequently need to access a variety of care services and providers at different stages in their supportive care journey. This can include primary, secondary, community and palliative care services. However, the varied communication pathways and networks between these different part of the healthcare infrastructure means that individuals can often fall through the cracks, due to assumptions that other care providers are supporting them. The mesothelioma specialist nurse can play a pivotal role in facilitating more joined-up communication between these different sectors by acting as the central point of contact for mesothelioma patients. This may help to reduce a sense of frustration at being bounced around the system without progress being made both by addressing supportive care needs and enhancing service efficiency.

Finally, collating a broader understanding of what works, for whom and in what context is key to assimilating crucial information that can inform how mesothelioma specialist nurses can be most effective in providing optimal care to people with mesothelioma and supporting them as they enter and move forward in their supportive cancer care pathways. This can help to make sure services are configured to accommodate the needs of people with mesothelioma, whilst also ensuring that they work well in terms of identifying the best working practices across different geographical settings, within a variety of healthcare services and systems. Ultimately, this can lead to enhanced supportive care that is delivered efficiently and effectively, for the benefit of people with mesothelioma.

REFERENCES

Ball, H., Moore, S. & Leary, A. (2016). A systematic literature review comparing the psychological care needs of patients with mesothelioma and advanced lung cancer. *European Journal of Oncology Nursing*, 25, pp. 62–67. https://doi.org/10.1016/j.ejon.2016.09.007

Davey, Z. & Henshall, C. (2021). Improving mesothelioma follow-up care in the UK: A qualitative study to build a multidisciplinary pyramid of care approach. *BMJ Open,* 11, p. e048394. https://doi.org/10.1136/bmjopen-2020-048394

de Boer, N.L. et al. (2019). Malignant peritoneal mesothelioma: patterns of care and survival in the Netherlands: A population-based study. *Annals of Surgical Oncology*, 26(13), pp. 4222–4228. https://doi.org/10.1245/s10434-019-07803-z

Ejegi-Memeh, S. (2022). Patients' and informal carers' experience of living with mesothelioma: A systematic rapid review and synthesis of the literature. *European Journal of Oncology Nursing*, 58, p. 102122. https://doi.org/10.1016/j.ejon.2022.102122.

Gardiner, C. et al. (2022). Clinical nurse specialist role in providing generalist and specialist palliative care: A qualitative study of mesothelioma clinical nurse specialists. *Journal of Advanced Nursing*, 78(9), pp. 2973–2982. https://doi.org/10.1111/jan.15277

Henshall C. et al. (2021). Recommendations for improving follow-up care for patients with mesothelioma: A qualitative study comprising documentary analysis, interviews and consultation meetings. *BMJ*, 11, p. e040679. https://doi.org/10.1136/bmjopen-2020-040679

Henshall C. et al. (2022). Understanding clinical decision-making in mesothelioma care: a mixed methods study. *BMJ Open Respiratory Research*, 9, p. e001312. https://doi.org/10.1136/bmjresp-2022-001312

Hoon, S.N., et al. (2021). Symptom burden and unmet needs in malignant pleural mesothelioma: Exploratory analyses from the RESPECT-Meso study. *Journal of Palliative Care*, 36(2), pp. 113–120. https://doi.org/10.1177/0825859720948975

Johnson, M., Allmark, P. & Tod, A. (2022). Living beyond expectations: A qualitative study into the experience of long-term survivors with pleural mesothelioma and their carers. *BMJ Open Respiratory research*, 9(1), p. e001252. https://doi.org/10.1136/bmjresp-2022-001252

Kerr, H., Donovan, M. & McSorley, O. (2021). Evaluation of the role of the clinical nurse specialist in cancer care: An integrative literature review. *European Journal of Cancer Care*, 30(3), e13415. https://doi.org/10.1111/ecc.13415

Kusamra, S. et al. (2021). Peritoneal mesothelioma: PSOGI/EURACAN clinical practice guidelines for diagnosis, treatment and follow-up. *European Journal of Surgical Oncology*, 47(1), pp. 36–59.

Lewis, R.A. et al. (2009). Patients' and healthcare professionals' views of cancer follow-up: Systematic review. *The British Journal of General Practice: The Journal of the Royal College of General Practitioners*, 59(564), pp. e248–e259. https://doi.org/10.3399/bjgp09X453576

Mesothelioma UK (2024). *Our Nurses*. Mesothelioma UK: Leicester. Available at: https://www.mesothelioma.uk.com/our-nurses/ (Accessed: 4 August 2024)

Sherborne, V. et al. (2020). What are the psychological effects of mesothelioma on patients and their carers? A scoping review. *Psycho-Oncology*, 29(10), pp. 1464–1473. https://doi.org/10.1002/pon.5454

Woolhouse, I., et al. (2018). British Thoracic Society guideline for the investigation and management of malignant pleural mesothelioma. *Thorax*, 73(Suppl 1), pp. i1–i30.

Chapter 8

Clinical trials

Bethany Taylor, Leah Taylor, Angela Tod and Simon Bolton

OVERVIEW

A clinical trial is research that studies a new intervention (e.g. a drug, device, procedure or service). A clinical trial will seek to understand whether the new intervention is more effective than existing treatment or care. It will establish how the intervention impacts on certain pre-specified outcomes, for example, quality of life or survival.

There are limited treatment options for people with mesothelioma. Therefore, clinical trials are vitally important as new interventions are developed, and need to be evaluated to see if they offer an improved treatment option for the future. However, access to mesothelioma clinical trials remains low. A recent survey conducted by Mesothelioma UK indicated 70% of patients had clinical trials discussed with them but only 36% participated.

This chapter will explore the role of clinical trials in the patient journey from the perspective of those experiencing them as a participant. As mesothelioma is an incurable condition, clinical trials may be the only way people can access a new treatment when standard treatment has failed. This creates challenges for the conduct of clinical trials.

In addition, there are a range of issues that influence how easy or possible it is for people to access and participate in a clinical trial if they have mesothelioma. These will be explained in the light of current evidence. Several issues can influence equitable access and create barriers and facilitators to accessing clinical trials. These include structural issues, factors related to healthcare professionals and finally, patient-focused factors that relate to the ability of someone to take part in a clinical trial. With reflections on current evidence, the chapter will consider patients' experiences of mesothelioma clinical trials from recruitment to participation, and after the clinical trial has finished.

DOI: 10.4324/9781032631318-8

The chapter finishes by considering the learning from existing evidence and presents key messages for practice relating to clinical trials in mesothelioma. The recommendations focus on good practice that helps people more easily access a clinical trial.

THE EVIDENCE

The role of clinical trials in mesothelioma

Clinical trials are conducted in phases: Phase I focuses on safety and dosage, Phase II on effectiveness and Phase III on comparing new treatments to the current standard of care. This rigorous process ensures that any new treatment approved for use is both safe for patients and more effective than existing options. In mesothelioma, clinical trials play a crucial role in testing new drugs, treatment combinations, and innovative approaches to care to improve treatments and patient outcomes, including enhanced survival and better quality of life. Despite some recent advancements in treatments, options remain limited. Some patients are too ill to endure the side effects of current treatments, highlighting the urgent need for new innovations. The rarity of mesothelioma complicates and lengthens recruitment for clinical trials. This delay is particularly troubling given the short life expectancy of many patients, as it can postpone the approval of new treatments until it is too late for current patients.

Trial design

Clinical trials are becoming increasingly complex in their design and procedures due to the demand for robust evidence and increasingly strict regulations for ethical and scientific trial conduct (Rodríguez-Torres et al., 2021). Health services research also must be conducted in a way that facilitates equality of access and inclusion, for example, for minority groups and people of any age and gender. There exists therefore an inbuilt challenge to balance the complexity with the need to make clinical trials easy to understand and accessible. For people with mesothelioma, understanding what a clinical trial is aiming to do and what it means for the participant may be additionally demanding. This is because of their pathway to a diagnosis and to trial recruitment. By the time someone is being considered for a trial they may have had a long and/or frightening pathway to diagnosis (see Chapter 4). In addition, they have had to receive, and try and understand, a high volume of information about mesothelioma, an incurable disease they may never have heard of before. To then process multifaceted information about clinical trials is especially demanding (Warnock et al., 2019).

Two concepts underpin many clinical trials in order to meet the need for scientific and ethical rigour: equipoise and randomisation. Equipoise exists when there is general uncertainty about the benefit or effectiveness of a drug or intervention. Randomisation is the process of allocating people to different groups in a clinical trial, for example, the trial drug (intervention) or current standard treatment (control group). The randomisation process means allocation is based on chance. Both these concepts are incredibly complicated to understand and become even more so when one considers the volume of information people with mesothelioma need to process when deciding whether to take part in a trial. Mesothelioma is a life-limiting condition making it sometimes difficult to process information about treatment and trial options. For some, current treatment may have been unsuccessful meaning access to a potential drug or procedure within a trial offers hope. For them, understanding or accepting equipoise and randomisation can be particularly challenging, especially if they have a preference for which arm of the trial they wish to be allocated to (Allmark & Tod, 2016). This was indicated in an interview-based sub-study of a recent randomised trial of surgery for pleural mesothelioma (Warnock et al., 2019).

A recent systematic review has identified 20 themes relating to barriers and facilitators to clinical trials, including factors relating to trial design and information. Personal experiences and attitudes, potential participant characteristics and culture were also found to play a role (Rodríguez-Torres et al., 2021). These factors highlight how increasingly hard it is to conduct clinical trials in mesothelioma that are accessible. Including patients and families in the co-production of trial design can be helpful (Warnock et al., 2019). In addition, conducting experience-based research within a clinical trial (often called nested studies), can provide insight into how trial designs can be improved to make them more acceptable to potential participants.

Barriers and facilitators to taking part in trials

Structural

It is possible to see, from the section above, how the complex structure of clinical trials can create barriers to people taking part. In addition, there are several structural barriers that impede people accessing clinical trials. In the main these barriers relate to the distance people have to travel, access to transport and conflicting responsibilities that would prevent travel.

As a rare disease, many people who develop mesothelioma may not live near a health centre or multidisciplinary team that specialises in mesothelioma. Not all clinical trials are open just in specialist centres. The chief investigator and lead site may be a specialist, but other hospitals may be involved in recruiting participants and even administering the trial intervention(s). However, where specialist knowledge and expertise are required for the trial, for example, where a new or specialist surgical technique is being evaluated, the study will be run in only a few centres. This was the case in the Mesothelioma and Radical Surgery 2 (MARS2) trial in the UK (Lim et al., 2024) and HIT-MESO (Hiley et al., 2024), a trial evaluating proton beam radiotherapy in mesothelioma. In trials such as these, participants may be faced with long journeys not only to receive the trial intervention, but also for pre-trial assessment and post-treatment follow-up and surveillance. Additional related barriers that have been cited include limited available parking, unreliable or complicated train journeys and having to stay overnight. All these problems have a knock-on financial implication, creating another structural barrier.

The impact of these factors, and the ability of a potential participant to overcome them, can be enhanced when the person is experiencing mesothelioma-related symptoms such as fatigue, breathlessness, pain, and emotional or psychological issues. People may decide against participating in the trial and focus instead on their current quality of life.

There is also potential for income-based inequality related to structural barriers. Where the cost of participation has financial consequences, people may have a further disincentive to participate. Some costs may be paid for through the trial. In the UK there are charitable funds that mesothelioma trial participants can apply for to cover the costs of participation, for example from Mesothelioma UK and various Asbestos Support Groups.

Factors relating to healthcare professionals.

Healthcare professionals are critical in enabling patients to make informed choices about their treatment and care including clinical trials. Health professionals can have a role in facilitating or creating barriers to recruitment and participation. However, who is the right person to discuss research with patients? Nurses are the largest workforce in the NHS and have a crucial role in many aspects of patient care; despite this, research has not been fully embedded in nursing roles (NHS England and NHS Improvement, 2021). In the past, research has been viewed by some nurses as the role of a doctor or a nurse working in a clinical research department. For many, research has been an area of limited knowledge steeped in intrigue and mystery. Also, patient information on clinical trials on current NHS websites advises talking to a doctor or a patient organisation about potential trial options. These factors contribute to an assumption that it is not necessarily a nursing role to discuss research participation. Lung cancer nurses are reported to be routinely called upon to discuss clinical trials with patients, yet it is acknowledged in the literature that they report concerns about their lack of education and training in this area (Lond et al., 2024). Nurses will be less inclined to discuss clinical trials with patients if they do not feel skilled to do so.

To feel empowered to discuss clinical trials with patients it is important to understand the aim of the treatment under investigation and the stage of the trial. There is a risk that clinical trials may be regarded by health professionals as futile, a last resort and something which should not replace standard treatment. This is particularly relevant to mesothelioma due to the high one-year mortality rate. The ATOMiC-Meso study compared doublet chemotherapy with and without the addition of a trial drug (Szlosarek et al., 2024). The intervention was shown to be beneficial to patients with certain types of mesothelioma. Despite this, patients were not always informed about this study even when they met the entry criteria for subtype, stage and fitness. Nihilistic attitudes may partially explain this.

Healthcare professionals may not be aware of other trials which exist outside of their centre and may not know how to find out. Clinical research websites can be confusing to navigate as the user must search and filter to bring up only current recruiting studies in the UK making it more of a challenge to find information easily during an already time limited patient consultation. The Mesothelioma UK clinical trials app lists information about location of current trials, treatment schedules and inclusion criteria (https://www.mesothelioma.uk.com/clinical-trials/). The information is written in plain language as far as possible to make it accessible for a wide audience. The information in the app is updated in real time which ensures it is current. The mesothelioma clinical nurse specialist (MCNS) team regularly receives educational updates about ongoing and forthcoming trials and is equipped to discuss participation with patients. Furthermore, investigators in the UK are aware of the unique network of the MCNSs and actively seek advice and guidance about possible recruitment sites in their area to ensure a good geographical distribution of trial centres. Several of the MCNSs are actively involved in clinical trials in their centres with some undertaking principal investigator roles on appropriate studies.

Factors relating to the person with mesothelioma.

Participating in a clinical trial is a multifaceted and complex decision. This section will consider motivations and obstacles to taking part from the perspective of the person with mesothelioma.

Motivation: Clinical trials offer access to cutting-edge treatments that are not yet available to the general public. Patients might be driven to take part by the hope and possibility that a new treatment could be more effective than existing standard treatments. This motivation is particularly strong among mesothelioma patients, given the poor prognosis of the disease and the hope for a clinical trial treatment to potentially be the long-awaited breakthrough.

Patients and carers who participated in the IRAMP study (Bolton et al., 2025) reported that for them, some clinical trials represented a potential new line of therapy when all other options had been exhausted. There was acknowledgement that they might not get a new drug or intervention within a trial and even if they did, it might not ultimately prove to be any better than current standard of care, yet the incentive was knowing that there was at least a potential of benefit for them as an individual.

> *"Taking part in research, the idea of that certainly appealed to me. I felt at least I was doing something."*

(Patient 2)

Another motivation to take part in clinical trials was the belief that they'd be helping others as well as themselves. One patient linked her participation to hope for others who'd be affected by the disease in the future.

> *"It's important for other people that are going to suffer with this in the future, that they've got a bit more hope and you've got to develop new drugs and new medication. And you can't do that without doing trials on human beings."*

(Patient 4)

Participants in a qualitative study embedded within the MARS2 clinical trial reported numerous reasons for their involvement. These included optimism, hope, altruism through contributing to medical research and helping future patients, a desire to receive the intervention and the additional support provided within the trial (Warnock et al., 2019). Clinical trial participation often entails increased surveillance due to additional monitoring, scans and interactions with healthcare professionals who have mesothelioma expertise, which can be reassuring. Other motivations include a determination to fight the disease, exhaustion of other treatment options or limited success with previous treatments, leading to a willingness to try anything. Long-term mesothelioma survivors highlighted their interest in clinical trials as a means to access otherwise unavailable treatments (Johnson et al., 2022). This motivation is complex because, in a clinical trial, patients are usually randomly allocated to either the new intervention or the standard treatment, meaning some participants may not receive the experimental treatment they hoped for.

Similar motivations to those mentioned here have been observed in other cancer patient groups (Nielsen & Berthelsen, 2019; Rodriguez-Torres et al, 2021).

Obstacles: Concerns about potential side effects, the inherent uncertainty of a clinical trial, lower tolerance for treatment or perceived limited benefits can lead individuals to opt out of clinical trials. Scepticism surrounding these trials and the association with being a "guinea pig" contribute to this. Additionally, for many patients, maintaining physical health and strength is a top priority. This concern, combined with the fear of side effects, can influence the decision to decline treatment for mesothelioma patients (Bibby et al., 2017).

Relatives are sometimes less enthusiastic about participating in a clinical trial compared to the patients themselves (Bibby et al., 2022). This may stem from a protective instinct or a desire to advocate on behalf of stoical patients. This highlights the differing concerns that relatives and patients may have, indicating the need for information and support for family members as well as patients.

Finally, some people choose not to take part in a clinical trial because of a lack of information about what is required and/or because the technical language used is difficult to understand (Rodriguez-Torres et al., 2021)

Expertise and trust in the clinical team: Access to healthcare professionals with specialist mesothelioma expertise is extremely valuable to patients. A recent study exploring access to clinical trials found that lack of specialist expertise restricted access (Bolton et al., 2025). The same study reported that having a health professional to act as an advocate for the patients, such as a mesothelioma CNS, facilitated trial access.

Trust in the medical team plays a crucial role in the decision-making process for patients. When healthcare professionals express a preference for certain treatment options, it can influence a patient's choice. Patients often seek certainty and reassurance from their healthcare providers, believing that their medical knowledge and expertise give them unique insights into the most effective treatment choices. This dynamic becomes particularly challenging in the context of equipoise within clinical trials, where the effectiveness of a treatment is uncertain – hence the necessity of conducting the trial. The qualitative study embedded within the MARS2 clinical trial demonstrated that healthcare professionals' attitudes towards the surgical intervention or clinical trials in general influenced patient engagement in the trial (Warnock et al., 2019). A more recent study (Bibby et al., 2022) illustrated how a patient's desire for certainty can affect their understanding of equipoise. One 61-year-old patient expressed frustration, saying:

> *"You know, one person says, 'It is not going to really do you a lot of good'. Another person says, 'Well, we don't know, it might do'. So, what do I do? I would rather somebody say, 'It is of no use to you whatsoever and don't bother' or, 'Go for it'. But don't wishy-washy in between either a yes or a no."*
> (Bibby et al., 2022, p. 5)

This study revealed that patients often believed healthcare professionals had insights into the clinical trial intervention and some assumed the intervention would be beneficial.

Practical issues that impact the decision about whether to participate in a clinical trial

The decision to participate in a clinical trial is multifaceted. Beyond the factors influencing a person's desire to enrol on a trial, several practical issues can shape and complicate this decision, including:

- *Financial costs*: Participation may incur direct costs such as accommodation if the trial hospital is far from home, as well as travel and parking expenses. Indirect financial implications might include a family member or friend taking time off work to accompany the patient.
- *Time and convenience*: The time commitment required for trial participation, including travel to the hospital and the frequency of visits, can affect willingness to participate. Patients with demanding personal or professional responsibilities may struggle to manage the logistics involved.
- *Trial availability*: There may not be a trial for which a patient is eligible or can travel to.
- *Access to non-NHS funded treatments*: Patients who have had a successful compensation claim may have funding for non-NHS treatments, allowing them to access additional treatment options without enrolling on a clinical trial.

Understanding the factors that facilitate and inhibit trial participation and impact upon patient experience of clinical trials is crucial for designing and conducting trials that are inclusive and patient centred. In return, this understanding has the potential to improve recruitment and retention rates. The evidence presented here raises questions about the inequities that inherently shape patient understanding of willingness and ability to partake in clinical trials.

Experiences during and after trials

Recruitment

Mesothelioma patients typically learn about clinical trials through online resources, their healthcare team or support groups. They may consider participating in a clinical trial shortly after diagnosis or at other stages in their treatment journey. The process of understanding trial information, including potential risks and benefits, can be overwhelming and often necessitates in-depth discussions with healthcare professionals. A study exploring people's experiences of surgery plus chemotherapy versus chemotherapy alone, the MARS2 clinical trial, has shown that it is challenging for patients to comprehend trial details shortly after diagnosis, as this is an emotionally distressing time when they are already processing a large amount of information (Warnock et al., 2019). As previously discussed, patients face various obstacles when considering clinical trial participation, many of which overlap with recruitment experiences, such as the difficulty in understanding complex trial information. Additionally, evidence indicates that the waiting period between consenting to participate and the actual start of the trial can be frustrating for patients (Warnock et al., 2019).

During the trial

Participation in a clinical trial for mesothelioma often requires patients to adhere to intensive treatment schedules, which include frequent hospital visits and numerous tests. Those randomised to the treatment arm may experience unpredictable side effects, leading to physical discomfort and impacts on their quality of life. While the uncertainty inherent in a clinical trial can offer hope, it can also cause significant anxiety. Regular assessments and monitoring can be reassuring for some patients, but for others, these frequent reminders of their disease can prevent them from engaging in activities they enjoy. Additionally, family commitments, such as caring responsibilities, can make it challenging for patients to attend the extra appointments.

The involvement of multiple care providers can lead to uncertainty and discontinuity in care (Warnock et al., 2019). For instance, if a patient experiences side effects, it may be unclear whether they should contact their usual local healthcare provider or the clinical trial team, creating confusion about the remit of each care provider. Participation in a clinical trial often necessitates travel to a hospital hosting the trial, which can be burdensome. For example, the HIT-MESO clinical trial, which began in 2024, involves proton beam therapy available at only two locations in the UK – Manchester and London. Patients randomised to receive this therapy must travel to these cities and undergo treatment over a five-week period. While free accommodation is provided for those who do not live nearby, some patients may be reluctant to stay away from home for this extended time.

A qualitative study on access to clinical trials for mesothelioma patients in Yorkshire (Bolton et al., 2025) reported that some patients had to travel considerable distances to participate, with one individual travelling over 100 miles from home.

For patients randomised to the control arm receiving standard treatment, experiences vary. Some accept this outcome, believing it to be the path meant for them, while others feel extreme disappointment and distress at not accessing the potentially better clinical trial treatment they had hoped for. Warnock et al. (2019) found that some participants remained in the MARS2 study even though they were not randomised to their preferred study arm. It is possible that this disappointment could lead to attrition, with some patients dropping out to enrol in another trial.

After the trial

Whilst people are participating in a clinical trial, they may not receive much care from their local or routine healthcare teams. Care, assessment and monitoring may be conducted by the research team. Trial participants often like this enhanced level of monitoring and health surveillance. However, it can create some concern after the trial ends. People may be unclear who is responsible for follow-up care and when it will be provided.

The MARS2 qualitative sub-study highlighted the need for careful transition of care from the clinical trial team to standard care delivered by the patient's local care provider (Warnock et al., 2019). If this is not done people can feel abandoned and alone when the additional monitoring and engagement with clinical trial healthcare professionals ends.

IMPLICATIONS FOR POLICY/PRACTICE

Recruitment to trials is a priority in order for new evidence-based treatments to be available for people with mesothelioma. To promote trial recruitment, it is essential that the factors driving patient motivation to take part are addressed and any obstacles they may face are reduced or overcome by improved trial design. This will serve to improve recruitment to future clinical trials.

There are elements of the trial design that can be modified to reduce participation barriers as outlined by Rodriguez-Torres et al. (2021). These include factors such as broadening eligibility criteria, using electronic communication to reduce site visits where possible, having more flexible hours for the participants' visits, reducing the number of visits required, using mobile medical professionals to visit participants at their location, reducing the trial duration and doing less intensive testing. Virtual Clinical Trials (VCT) have been proposed where trial activities are performed remotely using digital technologies. VCT does have potential, however, logistical problems can make them difficult to implement.

Strategies outlined here that can help in recruitment and decision-making regarding trial participation include incorporating trial recruitment into the CNS role, increased awareness and use of the Mesothelioma UK Clinical Trials app, and nationwide access to mesothelioma specialist MDTs.

Discussing clinical trials can be complex especially when, as in mesothelioma, a diagnosis is bewildering and difficult to understand. Alot of detail is needed to facilitate informed consent of trial participation because of ethical requirements. However, balancing this with information about the disease itself is difficult to achieve in a way that is accessible and acceptable to patients. Some CNSs will need training to be empowered to have conversations about research and trials. If appropriate, clinical trials need to be mentioned to patients as soon as possible. However, due to information overload, the discussion may need to be revisited in a timely manner. The CNS is well placed to do this.

Family members' information needs are often different to those of the person with mesothelioma. This should be acknowledged and the family's information needs incorporated through flexible service provision where appropriate and possible.

New ways to improve experiences of people during a trial and afterwards need to be developed. This includes addressing logistical issues like travel and cost as well as clear messaging about how to access help and from whom, for example, who to contact regarding treatment side effects, and what happens after a trial ends.

REFERENCES

Allmark, P. & Tod, A.M. (2016). Ethical challenges in conducting clinical research in lung cancer. *Translational Lung Cancer Research*, 5(3), pp. 219–226. https://doi.org/10.21037/tlcr.2016.03.04.

Bibby, A.C. et al. (2017). Exploring the characteristics of patients with mesothelioma who chose active treatment symptom control over chemotherapy as first line treatment: A prospective observational single centre study. *BMC Palliative Care*, 16(71). https://doi.org/10.1186/s12904-017-0255-3

Bibby, A.C. et al. (2022). The priorities of people with mesothelioma and their carers: A qualitative interview study of trial participation and treatment decisions. *European Journal of Oncology Nursing*, 57. https://doi.org/10.1016/j.ejon.2022.102111

Bolton, S., Lusted, C., Taylor, B. & Tod, A. (2025). *Improving Research Access for Mesothelioma Patients (IRAMP)*. 23rd British Thoracic Oncology Group Annual Conference 2025. 3rd–5th March 2025. Belfast. (Unpublished at date of writing)

Hiley, C. et al. (2024), P4.14C.08 HIT-MESO: Hemithoracic Irradiation with Proton Therapy in Malignant Pleural Mesothelioma. UK National Proton Radiotherapy Study. *Journal of Thoracic Oncology*, 19(10), p. S411.

Johnson, M., Allmark, P. & Tod A. (2022). Living beyond expectations: A qualitative study into the experience of long-term survivors with pleural mesothelioma and their carers. *BMJ Open Respiratory Research*, 9(1). https://doi.org/10.1136/bmjresp-2022-001252

Lim, E. et al. (2024). Extended pleurectomy decortication and chemotherapy versus chemotherapy alone for pleural mesothelioma (MARS 2): A phase 3 randomised controlled trial. *The Lancet*, 12(6), pp. 457–466. https://doi.org/10.1016/S2213-2600(24)00119-X

Lond, B. et al. (2024). A systematic review of the barriers and facilitators impacting patient enrolment in clinical trials for lung cancer. *European Journal of Oncology Nursing*, 70(102564). https://doi.org/10.1016/j.ejon.2024.102564

Nielsen, Z.E. & Berthelsen, C.B. (2019). Cancer patients' perceptions of factors influencing their decisions on participation in clinical drug trials: A qualitative meta-synthesis. *Journal of Clinical Nursing*, 28, pp. 2443–2461. https://doi.org/10.1111/jocn.14785.

NHS England and NHS Improvement (2021). *Chief Nursing Officer for England Strategic plan*. NHS England and NHS Improvement. Available at: https://www.england.nhs.uk/wp-content/uploads/2021/11/B0880-cno-for-englands-strategic-plan-fo-research.pdf (Accessed: September 2024)

Rodríguez-Torres, E., González-Pérez, M.M. & Díaz-Pérez, C. (2021) Barriers and facilitators to the participation of subjects in clinical trials: An overview of reviews. *Contemporary Clinical Trials Communications*, 23(100829). https://doi.org/10.1016/j.conctc.2021.100829

Szlosarek, PW. et al. (2024). ATOMIC-Meso Study Group. Pegargiminase plus first-line chemotherapy in patients with non epithelioid pleural mesothelioma: The ATOMIC-Meso randomized clinical trial. *JAMA Oncology*, 10(4), pp. 475–483. https://doi.org/10.1001/jamaoncol.2023.6789

Warnock, C. et al. (2019). Patient experiences of participation in a radical thoracic surgical trial: Findings from the Mesothelioma and Radical Surgery Trial 2 (MARS 2). *Trials*, 20(598). https://doi.org/10.1186/s13063-019-3692-x

Chapter 9

Palliative and end-of-life care in mesothelioma

Clare Gardiner and Sarah Hargreaves

OVERVIEW

In this chapter we explore key issues relating to palliative and end-of-life care in mesothelioma, with a particular focus on the UK context. We begin by providing definitions of key terms such as palliative care and end-of-life care and highlight the evidence base for a palliative care approach. In the UK, a range of different healthcare professionals are involved in providing palliative care, and we outline the role of generalist and specialist palliative care providers, in particular focusing on the palliative care role of mesothelioma clinical nurse specialists. The role of Asbestos Support Groups, legal companies and the charity Mesothelioma UK is discussed, particularly their role in providing benefits advice and support groups. End-of-life care in mesothelioma is then examined, looking at the limited evidence on where people with mesothelioma die, and providing an overview of end-of-life experiences from the perspectives of families. The chapter then explores barriers to accessing palliative care, including negative perceptions by patients and families. Finally, we describe a range of resources that have been developed in response to research findings from the Mesothelioma UK Research Centre to address some of the identified gaps in care. The chapter concludes by outlining implications and recommendations for practice and policy.

THE EVIDENCE

Palliative care needs in mesothelioma

Palliative care has an important role in mesothelioma, and people with mesothelioma and their families have palliative care needs from diagnosis to the end of life. While many different definitions exist for the term "palliative care" here we use the World

DOI: 10.4324/9781032631318-9

Health Organisation (WHO) definition which describes "a care approach to improve the quality of life of patients and that of their families who are facing challenges associated with life-threatening illness" (WHO, 2020). The terms palliative care and end-of-life care are often used synonymously, but a clear distinction is helpful for care delivery and for patient engagement. The UK charity Marie Curie defines "end of life care" as an approach that provides treatment and support for people who are near the end of their life, usually those who are thought to be in the last year of their life. Palliative care may include end-of-life care, but typically involves earlier engagement and broader considerations of quality of life, which are crucial in mesothelioma (Marie Curie, 2024). Internationally definitions may differ, but here we focus on the UK context. Evidence from a wide range of conditions has consistently shown that palliative care improves the quality of life of patients with palliative care needs and leads to improved outcomes for patients and their families (Smith et al., 2014; Bajwah 2020).

Mesothelioma has a poor prognosis. In the majority of cases the condition progresses rapidly, and most people will die within one to two years of diagnosis. Those who do survive longer often have complex needs and may have periods with high symptom burden. As a consequence, people with mesothelioma and their families have palliative care needs throughout the relatively short trajectory of their illness (Tinkler et al., 2017). People with mesothelioma experience a range of complex and debilitating symptoms which give rise to palliative care needs including fatigue, dyspnoea, pain, cough, weight loss, anxiety, low mood and anhedonia (Hoon et al., 2021). A 2021 integrative systematic review provides the most comprehensive account of palliative care needs in mesothelioma. The authors reported needs across a range of dimensions including organisation and co-ordination of services, communication and information needs, management of care needs and high symptom burden and consideration of the impact of seeking compensation. They concluded that the needs of patients and carers are underpinned by a pervasive sense of uncertainty, particularly relating to the progression of the disease within the context of a rare and terminal cancer (Harrison et al., 2021).

Compared with other cancers, the palliative care needs of people with mesothelioma and their families are particularly challenging to manage due to the complexity of symptoms which are often difficult to palliate, the rapidity of decline, and the asbestos causation which is associated with lengthy legal and compensation claims and the need for a coroner's inquiry (Harrison et al., 2021). Patients with mesothelioma often face distinct psychological challenges, including posttraumatic stress, due to the preventable causation (Sherborne et al., 2024). Due to the rarity of the condition health professionals often have limited expertise in mesothelioma management and in addressing the specific palliative care needs of mesothelioma patients and their families.

Family and other unpaid carers of patients with mesothelioma can have their own distinct palliative care needs, yet carers' needs are often neglected or left unaddressed. A 2022 qualitative interview study of bereaved mesothelioma carers found that they expressed needs around preparedness for "what lies ahead" and honest communication with health professionals (Harrison et al., 2022). Particular challenges have been noted with bereavement and coping after the death of the patient, with some carers describing a lack of insight into grief and feelings of abandonment after the patient has died (Harrison et al., 2022). Other studies have suggested that carers often put their own needs aside, in order to try and "stay strong" in front of the patient (Prusak et al., 2021).

Who provides palliative care in mesothelioma?

The role of palliative care in mesothelioma has been highlighted in UK and international clinical guidance. The British Thoracic Society guideline for the investigation and management of malignant pleural mesothelioma recommends the "early involvement of palliative care specialists" (Woolhouse et al., 2018). Guidance from the National Lung Cancer Forum for Nurses highlights the important role nurses play in the provision of palliative care and suggests that a range of supportive and palliative care specialist interventions can be used by healthcare professionals (Richardson et al., 2013). The European Respiratory Society guidance for the management of mesothelioma makes limited reference to palliative care, but does acknowledge the role of specialist palliative care in pain control and other physical symptoms (Scherpereel et al., 2010).

Both specialist and generalist palliative care are important in the care of patients with mesothelioma, offering distinct but complementary approaches to care. Specialist palliative care (SPC) is defined as care provided by those who have specialist training or expertise in palliative care, such as palliative medicine consultants and clinical nurse specialists in palliative care. Generalist palliative care is defined as care provided by any health and social care professionals who are not part of a specialist palliative care team and is a care approach that should be available throughout the course of a life-limiting illness (Robinson et al., 2022). An integrated approach to the provision of palliative care recognises the roles and responsibilities of both generalist and specialist palliative care providers and is increasingly advocated in order to provide comprehensive care (Gardiner et al., 2012).

Studies of palliative care in mesothelioma are sparse, however, in 2019 a multicentre randomised controlled trial in the UK and Australia (the RESPECT trial) explored early referral to SPC in malignant pleural mesothelioma. In this study early palliative care did not lead to any improvements in quality of life when compared with standard care, although a benefit in carer quality of life was noted (Brims et al., 2019). The authors hypothesised that current standards of palliative care management in the UK and Australia were already sufficient to meet patients' early palliative care needs (Brims et al., 2019) and therefore early SPC did not confer any additional benefit. In the UK, current standards of palliative care management in mesothelioma include substantial care provision from Mesothelioma UK clinical nurse specialists (MCNS). MCNSs provide specialist support and care to people living with mesothelioma and their families, including providing palliative and end-of-life care. A recent study exploring the MCNS role in mesothelioma found palliative care was perceived as integral to the MCNS role, and joint working with specialist palliative care and community services was required to provide holistic care. However, negative perceptions and misconceptions of palliative care services among patients were widely acknowledged by MCNSs and were seen as a barrier to patients accepting palliative care (Gardiner et al., 2022b).

Whilst mesothelioma clinical nurse specialists are known to improve palliative care provision for patients and carers (Gardiner et al., 2022a; 2022b), the availability of MCNSs is not uniform across the UK, and in some areas patients with mesothelioma will have no access to an MCNS (Wakefield et al., 2024). In the absence of a mesothelioma specialist nurse, most patients will have access to a lung cancer specialist nurse (for pleural mesothelioma) or other specialist nurse (for peritoneal and other types of mesotheliomas). Evidence suggests these nurses similarly have an important role in palliative care, and have experience of symptom control, but may lack specialist expertise in mesothelioma (Osborne & Kerr, 2021). Whilst specialist nurses have an integral role in palliative care, an integrated palliative care approach in mesothelioma involves a wide range of health and social care professionals from across the multidisciplinary team (MDT), specialist palliative care and primary care. Although this model has been widely advocated, evidence suggests challenges with implementing a truly integrated palliative care approach, including fragmentation of care, deskilling of generalist providers and difficulties with equitable use of limited specialist resources (Quill & Abernethy, 2013).

The charitable sector is also a key provider of palliative care support for mesothelioma patients and their families. The UK national charity Mesothelioma UK, for example, provides a wealth of information and support services including information about palliative care needs, end-of-life care and benefits advice to ensure that families receive the financial support they are entitled to. Patients, families and healthcare professionals can access support from an MCNS via Mesothelioma UK's free telephone support line, or email. This service is particularly important to patients and families without access to an MCNS in their locality. In addition, Mesothelioma UK and the UK-wide network of Asbestos

Support Groups provide both face-to-face and online support group meetings. Opportunities to meet with other people sharing similar experiences can be helpful both in sharing and gaining information and emotional support, and in helping people feel less alone (Breen et al., 2022; Ejegi-Memeh et al., 2021; 2024). However, some patients do not feel comfortable discussing palliative care issues in a support group setting, and they may not meet everyone's needs (Hoon et al., 2021, Sherborne et al., 2024).

The role of legal companies in helping people seek compensation for asbestos exposure is a unique part of palliative care support in mesothelioma (Harrison et al., 2021). The process of seeking compensation can be burdensome, coming at a time when patients and families are facing a devastating prognosis, and for whom time may be limited (Ball et al., 2016). However, financial redress can provide some comfort for people with mesothelioma in knowing that their families will be supported after their death (Ball et al., 2016; Ejegi-Memeh et al., 2024). A further positive aspect of the legal process is the supportive relationships that can develop between legal professionals and mesothelioma families. Legal teams can spend considerable amounts of time with patients and their families, and for many this is a cathartic and supportive interaction. However, compensation cases can be protracted, and the act of seeking compensation from former employers can give rise to complex emotions (Guglielmucci et al., 2018; Sherborne et al., 2024). Cases that are not resolved during the lifetime of the person with mesothelioma provide an additional burden and source of distress for bereaved families (Harrison et al., 2022; Sherborne et al., 2024).

End-of-life care in mesothelioma

There is a paucity of published evidence on where people with mesothelioma die. This is due to the rarity of mesothelioma which means published statistics on deaths generally relate to broader disease categories, e.g. lung cancer. In addition, there is limited research evidence on experiences of end-of-life care in mesothelioma. Published research identifies gaps in end-of-life care within the home setting due to a lack of preparedness and information (Harrison et al., 2022), poorly managed pain and a lack of required equipment (Lee et al., 2022). Poor end-of-life experiences can result in families suffering trauma after witnessing uncontrolled pain and distress in their loved one, which in turn can lead to prolonged and complex grief (Sherborne et al., 2024; Nagamatsu et al., 2022) (see Chapter 10 for further information).

Recent research from the Mesothelioma UK Research Centre found evidence of major gaps in end-of-life care (Harrison 2022; MURC, 2024). Participants frequently described disjointed care and a lack of advanced planning by healthcare professionals. In many instances a sudden decline in health led to families discovering at a very late stage that end of life was imminent; and in some cases families were uninformed and lost the opportunity to be present at end of life. The quality of care varied, however, the majority of participants recounted poor experiences, particularly in the hospital setting. Within the home setting there were repeated accounts of families being uninformed about what a death at home entails for the family, and in particular that support and care from healthcare professionals would be intermittent and there would be gaps in care (for further information see Chapter 10: The legacy of mesothelioma on families).

What are the gaps in palliative and end-of-life care?

Whilst encouraging progress has been made in the provision of palliative care in mesothelioma, in part as a consequence of the developing evidence base, some gaps in care provision remain. Mesothelioma poses many unique challenges which can hamper a palliative care approach. It is a rare cancer typified by a rapid decline and complex symptomatology, patients are more likely to suffer from intractable progressive pain and recurrent pleural effusions than those with lung cancer (Clayson et al., 2005). The pathophysiology of pain in mesothelioma makes it extremely challenging to treat, and it often requires multiple different types of analgesia (Macloed et al., 2015). Psychological distress can also be more severe than other types of cancer, and family carer needs may be greater due to the preventable causation and associated legal issues (Harrison et al., 2022).

Further barriers to timely access to palliative care include patient and family factors. Patients with mesothelioma and their families can be reluctant to accept palliative care due to misconceptions about the purpose of such care. Fear, stigma and negative connotations associated with palliative care services can result in delayed access to vital services for some patients (Gardiner et al., 2022b). In a survey of over 500 patients with mesothelioma, 63% stated that support from a palliative care nurse "had not been needed" and 73% reported not needing any support in relation to end-of-life planning, despite reporting considerable challenges with managing physical and psychological symptoms (Gardiner et al., 2022a). Societal stigma and public attitudes to death and dying have undoubtedly contributed to such reluctance to accept palliative care, and a significant proportion of UK adults report being uncomfortable discussing death and dying with family and friends (Dying Matters Coaltion, 2016). Targeted information provision relaying the benefits of palliative care in mesothelioma, and addressing misconceptions about such care, is an important step in addressing this information gap.

Access to palliative care may also be influenced by availability of services, inconsistent referral criteria, and local variations in organisation and delivery of treatment and care. A 2022 study found that referrals to specialist palliative care were often delayed due to "bottlenecks" in the system and were hampered by a lack of specialist mesothelioma knowledge amongst referring clinicians (Gardiner et al., 2022b). Evidence suggests that generalist care is likely to constitute the mainstay of palliative care in mesothelioma, with an important role for clinical nurse specialists (particularly MCNSs) and primary care (Gardiner et al., 2022a). Collaboration and communication with specialist palliative care is crucial in order to support patients with the most complex needs, however gaps in care persist and some patients are not well supported at the end of life (Gardiner et al., 2022b).

Palliative care resources to support patients, families and professionals

In order to address barriers to timely engagement with palliative care and the challenges faced by healthcare professionals who may be unfamiliar with this rare cancer, in 2023 a range of resources were developed Mesothelioma UK Research Centre (MURC) using a co-production approach. Researchers from MURC worked together with a creative design company, the charity Mesothelioma UK and the MURC patient and public involvement (PPI) panel. The following resources were developed:

1 **Palliative care animation and infographic**
   The three-minute animation is aimed at patients and families. It explains what palliative care is, addresses misunderstandings and outlines the benefits of early-stage engagement. The animation is freely available from the Mesothelioma UK website (MURC Co-production, 2023) and can be used as a resource to signpost patients and families, or as a means of opening conversations about palliative care.
      The key messages of the animation have been distilled into a one-page infographic which is also freely available (MURC Co-production, 2023).
2 **Healthcare professional infographic**
   A one-page infographic provides key information about palliative care needs and management in mesothelioma. It is aimed primarily at primary care healthcare professionals who may be unfamiliar with mesothelioma due to the rarity of the condition (Hargreaves et al., 2022; 2023). The infographic signposts to sources of further information available from the charity Mesothelioma UK. (MURC Co-production, 2023).
3 **Online event "Conversations about palliative care"**
   An online event held in 2023 featured as part of the Economic and Social Sciences Research Council (ESRC) Festival of Social Sciences. It brought

together researchers, mesothelioma patients and carers, and palliative care healthcare professionals to talk about what palliative care is, what are the misunderstandings and how palliative care can help both patients and families. It is freely available to view (MURC Event 2023).

IMPLICATIONS FOR POLICY/PRACTICE

The evidence presented here has important implications for palliative care provision in mesothelioma, recommendations for clinical practice and policy include:

- Addressing barriers to palliative care provision by increasing awareness, amongst clinicians, of the palliative care needs of patients with mesothelioma and their families.
- Acknowledging the crucial role of clinical nurse specialists in providing palliative care, and embedding a palliative care approach within the job specification for all CNSs involved in mesothelioma care, particularly mesothelioma CNSs.
- Developing and implementing strategies to address misconceptions about palliative care amongst patients with mesothelioma and their families, for example, by utilising the resources described above to open conversations about palliative care.
- Consider adopting a broader public health approach to palliative care in order to engage communities and citizens in supporting palliative care needs among patients with mesothelioma and their families.
- Ensuring that both patients and families are aware of the range of support services available, and in particular the different options available to meet with other people living through similar experiences.
- Acknowledging the burden experienced by patients and families going through the compensation process, with an awareness that experiences vary and processes can be protracted and emotionally demanding.
- Improving access to advance care planning for patients and families to ensure choices around end of life are informed and take account of needs.

Patients with mesothelioma and their families need skilled and timely palliative care support to enable them to live well and maximise quality of life. Good palliative care should be a fundamental component of care and support for any mesothelioma patient, yet many never receive this care and suffer profoundly as a consequence. By reframing palliative care as the responsibility of the whole multidisciplinary team, patients and their families can benefit from a palliative care approach from diagnosis to the end of life. The crucial role of clinical nurse specialists also requires further recognition, as core providers of palliative care and experts in the complexities of mesothelioma. Palliative care in mesothelioma goes beyond the health workforce, and patients can be supported by others including charities, legal firms and support groups. Finally, wider public misunderstandings about palliative care and societal stigma surrounding dying have contributed to negative perceptions of palliative care. Ongoing work to engage not only the mesothelioma community, but also the wider public, in conversations about death and dying are an important step in addressing this.

REFERENCES

Ball, H., Moore, S. & Leary, A. (2016). A systematic literature review comparing the psychological care needs of patients with mesothelioma and advanced lung cancer. *European Journal of Oncology Nursing*, 25, pp. 62–67.

Brims. F., et al. (2019). Early specialist palliative care on quality of life for malignant pleural mesothelioma: a randomised controlled trial. *Thorax*, 74(4), pp. 354–361.

Bajwah, S., Oluyase, A.O., Yi, D., Gao, W., Evans, C.J., Grande, G., Todd, C., Costantini, M., et al. (2020). The effectiveness and cost-effectiveness of hospital-based specialist palliative care for adults with advanced illness and their caregivers. *Cochrane Database of Systematic Reviews*, (9). https://doi.org/10.1002/14651858.CD012780.pub2

Breen, L.J., Huseini, T., Same, A., Peddle-McIntyre, C.J. & Lee, Y.G. (2022). Living with mesothelioma: A systematic review of patient and caregiver psychosocial support needs. *Patient Education and Counseling*, 105(7), pp.1904–1916.

Clayson, H., Seymour, J. & Noble, B. (2005). Mesothelioma from the patient's perspective. *Hematology/Oncology Clinics*, 19(6), pp. 1175–1190.

Dying Matters Coalition (2016). *Public opinion on death and dying*. Available at: https://www.dyingmatters.org/sites/default/files/files/NCPC_Public%20polling%2016_Headline%20findings_1904.pdf

Ejegi-Memeh, S., Robertson, S., Taylor, B., Darlison, L. & Tod, A. (2021). Gender and the experiences of living with mesothelioma: A thematic analysis. *European Journal of Oncology Nursing*, 52, p. 101966.

Ejegi-Memeh, S., Sherborne, V., Mayland, C., Tod, A. & Taylor, B.H. (2024). Mental health and wellbeing in mesothelioma: A qualitative study exploring what helps the wellbeing of those living with this illness and their informal carers. *European Journal of Oncology Nursing*, 70, p. 102572.

Gardiner, C., Gott, M. & Ingleton, C. (2012). Factors supporting good partnership working between generalist and specialist palliative care services: A systematic review. *British Journal of General Practice*, 62(598), pp. 252–253.

Gardiner, C., Harrison, M., Hargreaves, S. & Taylor, B. (2022a). Palliative care roles and responsibilities of mesothelioma clinical nurse specialists in the UK. *Progress in Palliative Care*. https://doi.org/10.1080/09699260.2022.2158286

Gardiner C., Harrison M., Hargreaves S. & Taylor B. (2022b). Clinical nurse specialist role in providing generalist and specialist palliative care: A qualitative study of mesothelioma clinical nurse specialists. *Journal of Advanced Nursing*, 00, pp. 1–10. https://doi.org/10.1111/jan.15277

Guglielmucci, F., Franzoi, I.G., Bonafede, M., Borgogno, F.V., Grosso, F. & Granieri, A. (2018). "The less I think about it, the better I feel": A thematic analysis of the subjective experience of malignant mesothelioma patients and their caregivers. *Frontiers in Psychology*, 9, p. 320693.

Hargreaves, S., Gardiner, C., & Couchman, E. (2022). Caring for mesothelioma patients and their families in primary care: New tools to enable early-stage engagement with palliative care. GP Life, Available at: https://bjgplife.com/caring-for-mesothelioma-patients-and-their-families-in-primary-care-new-tools-to-enable-early-stage-engagement-with-palliative-care/ (Accessed: June 2024)

Hargreaves, S., Gardiner, C., Tod, A. & Darlison, L. (2023). Mesothelioma palliative care needs: Supporting patients and families with new research-based resources. *British Journal of Community Nursing*, 28(5), pp. 248–252.

Harrison, M., Gardiner, C., Taylor, B., Ejegi-Memeh, S. & Darlison, L. (2121). Understanding the palliative care needs and experiences of people with mesothelioma and their family carers: An integrative systematic review. *Palliative Medicine*, 35(6), pp. 1039–1051.

Harrison, M., Darlison, L. & Gardiner, C. (2022). Understanding the experiences of end of life care for patients with mesothelioma from the perspective of bereaved family caregivers in the UK: A qualitative analysis. *Journal of Palliative Care*, February. https://doi.org/10.1177/08258597221079235

Hoon, S.N., Lawrie, I., Qi, C., Rahman, N., Maskell, N., Forbes, K., Gerry, S., Monterosso, L., et al. (2021). Symptom burden and unmet needs in malignant pleural mesothelioma: Exploratory analyses from the RESPECT-Meso study. *Journal of Palliative Care*, 36(2), pp. 113–120. https://doi.org/10.1177/0825859720948975

Lee, J.T., Mittal, D.L., Warby, A., Kao, S., Dhillon, H.M. & Vardy JL. (2022). Dying of mesothelioma: A qualitative exploration of caregiver experiences. *European Journal of Cancer Care*, 31(5), p. e13627.

MacLeod, N., Klepstad, P., Fallon, M. & Laird, B. (2015). Pain management in mesothelioma. *Reports of Radiotherapy and Oncology*, 2(3).

Marie Curie (2024). *What is end of life care?* Available at: https://www.mariecurie.org.uk/help/support/terminal-illness/preparing/end-of-life-care (Accessed: 20 May 2024)

Mesothelioma UK Research Centre (MURC). *Supporting Our Supporters (SoS)*. Available at: https://www.sheffield.ac.uk/murc/supporting-our-supporters (Accessed: 20 November 2024)

Mesothelioma UK Research Centre (MURC) Co-production (2023). *Mesothelioma palliative care resources*. Available at: https://www.mesothelioma.uk.com/palliative-care/ (patient/family webpage); https://www.mesothelioma.uk.com/for-healthcare-professionals/palliative-care/ (healthcare professional webpage) (Accessed: June 2024)

Mesothelioma UK Research Centre (MURC) Event (2023). *Conversations about palliative care*. Available at: https://player.sheffield.ac.uk/events/conversations-about-palliative-care (Accessed: June 2024)

Nagamatsu, Y., Sakyo, Y., Barroga, E., Koni, R., Natori, Y. & Miyashita, M. (2022). Depression and complicated grief, and associated factors, of bereaved family members of patients who died of malignant pleural mesothelioma in Japan. *Journal of Clinical Medicine*, 11(12), p. 3380. https://doi.org/10.3390/jcm11123380

Osborne, J. & Kerr, H. (2021). Role of the clinical nurse specialist as a non-medical prescriber in managing the palliative care needs of individuals with advanced lung cancer. *International Journal of Palliative Nursing*, 27(4), pp. 205–212. https://doi.org/10.12968/ijpn.2021.27.4.205

Prusak, A., van der Zwan, J.M., Aarts, M.J., Arber, A., Cornelissen, R., Burgers, S., & Duijts, S.F.A. (2021). The psychosocial impact of living with mesothelioma: Experiences and needs of patients and their carers regarding supportive care. *European Journal of Cancer Care*, 30(6), p. e13498.

Quill, T.E. & Abernethy, A.P. (2013). Generalist plus specialist palliative care – creating a more sustainable model. *New England Journal of Medicine*, 368(13), pp. 1173–1175. https://doi.org/10.1056/NEJMp1215620

Richardson, A., Draffan, J. & White J. (2013). 117 National Lung Cancer Forum For Nurses Supported By Lilly Project 2011/2012 – Developing guidance for the supportive and palliative care of lung cancer and mesothelioma patients and their carers. *Nursing & Supportive Care*, 79(Suppl 1), pp. S40–S41.

Robinson, J., Frey, R., Raphael, D., Old, A. & Gott, M. (2022). Difficulties in navigating the intersection of generalist and specialist palliative care services: A cross-sectional study of bereaved family's experiences of care at home in New Zealand. *Health and Social Care in the Community*, 30, pp. 133–141. https://doi.org/10.1111/hsc.13381

Scherpereel, A., et al. (2010). Guidelines of the European Respiratory Society and the European Society of Thoracic Surgeons for the management of malignant pleural mesothelioma. *European Respiratory Society*, 35, pp. 479–495.

Sherborne, V., Wood, E., Mayland, C., Gardiner, C., Lusted, C., Bibby, A., Tod, A., Taylor, B., et al. (2024). The mental health and well-being implications of a mesothelioma diagnosis: A mixed methods study. *European Journal of Oncology Nursing*. Available online 15 March 2024, 102545. https://doi.org/10.1016/j.ejon.2024.102545

Smith, S., Brick, A., O'Hara, S. & Normand, C. (2014). Evidence on the cost and cost-effectiveness of palliative care: A literature review. Palliative Medicine, 28(2), pp. 130–150.

Tinkler, M., Royston, R. & Kendall C. (2017). Palliative care for patients with mesothelioma. *British Journal of Hospital Medicine*, 78, pp. 219–225.

Wakefield, D., Ward, T., Edge, H., Mayland, C.R. & Gardiner, C. (2024). Too little, too late? Patients & families with mesothelioma experience unmet care needs, even after death. *Palliative Medicine*, 38, (1) (Suppl: 2024 EAPC WR CongressMar 2024), pp. 1–280).

World Health Organisation (WHO). 2020. *Factsheet: Palliative care*. Available at: https://www.who.int/news-room/fact-sheets/detail/palliative-care (Accessed: 20 May 2024)

Woolhouse, I., Bishop, L., Darlison, L., et al. (2018). BTS guideline for the investigation and management of malignant pleural mesothelioma. *Thorax*, 73(Suppl 1), p. 2

Chapter 10

The legacy of the illness for the family

Sarah Hargreaves, Sarah Thomas and Samantha Cox

OVERVIEW

This chapter describes how family experiences during the course of the illness, at end of life and in the period after the death create a distinctive legacy for mesothelioma families. Mesothelioma is a preventable and incurable condition caused by exposure to asbestos. Families live with this knowledge and the profound emotional impact of the disease. This is core to the family legacy of the illness.

This chapter focuses on different time points in family experiences and how they shape the family legacy. We begin by describing experiences during the course of the illness and their impact on bereavement, such as, the differing trajectories experienced in mesothelioma (e.g. a late-stage diagnosis and rapid decline). End-of-life experiences vary for families and can be challenging due to the complexity and severity of mesothelioma symptoms. We present research evidence exploring both positive and negative experiences and the implications for bereavement.

When someone with mesothelioma dies the coroner (or procurator fiscal in Scotland) has to investigate because in most cases the death is not due to natural causes; it is mainly due to occupational asbestos exposure and is classified as an industrial disease. The coronial/procurator fiscal procedures within the UK are described, and the impact on families of inquest at a time of grief.

The chapter ends with an exploration of support needs in bereavement; and concludes with recommendations and implications for practice to better support families living with the legacy of mesothelioma.

DOI: 10.4324/9781032631318-10

THE EVIDENCE

Experiences across the disease trajectory

Whilst mesothelioma is experienced directly by the person with mesothelioma, families experience the disease trajectory alongside their relatives. The devastating impact is captured by Lee et al. (2022) where a participant stated that the family "all lived" the disease. Diagnosis is described as a time of shock. The predominant memory is often of being told that mesothelioma is incurable, and that time is short. This negative experience can have a lasting impact on families (Lee et al., 2022; Sherborne et al., 2024b; Taylor et al., 2019). This defining experience puts pressure on families to both support their relatives and make the most of this time within a compressed and uncertain future. Different methods of communicating the diagnosis by healthcare professionals can alter family perceptions of this traumatic event, for example, if the diagnosis is conveyed in a way that stresses the support available and the individual nature of mesothelioma journeys, these positive aspects can be recalled when looking back at the diagnosis (Sherborne et al., 2024b). Case studies of patients with cancer identified that when bad news is given, patients and their families hear it through different filters (Hottensen, 2010). Whilst the patient and their family can be in the same room and hear the same diagnosis, it can be an entirely different experience. There are many strong emotions which may arise, including shock, disbelief, fear, anger and sadness.

A preventable death

Mesothelioma is a preventable condition, which adds to the shock and emotional impact at diagnosis. It is important to understand the role that anger plays within mesothelioma (Ejegi-Memeh et al., 2024). Triggers for this emotion may include: a prolonged diagnostic journey, a short prognosis, possibility of rapid deterioration, loss of future plans and feelings of injustice. It is essential that mental health professionals recognise that underneath anger there is always pain. Therefore, a safe environment must be created, which can help give hope when the future seems uncertain.

Anticipatory grief

Due to the time lag between asbestos exposure and the development of mesothelioma, the diagnosis occurs typically in retirement. Retirement plans are abandoned, and couples in very long-term partnerships face the loss of a life partner. Anticipatory grief is common (Sherborne et al., 2024b). In the recent study Supporting our Supporters (SoS), which explored the experiences of family supporting relatives living with mesothelioma, participants living in long-term partnerships spoke of their fears for the future, and dread of being alone. This experience of anticipatory grief is replicated in Gibson et al.'s study (2024).

CS Lewis described his grief saying that *"no one ever told me that grief felt so like fear"* (Goodreads, 2016). The threat of loss may set in motion the grieving process for the patient with mesothelioma and their families. Worden (1983) describes this process of grieving before the actual loss as anticipatory grief. Mental health professionals can help identify the series of losses for both the patient and their family. These may include, for example, change in relationships and loss of roles, affection, physical health and independence. The loss of roles may include an individual losing the physical capacity to mow the lawn, resulting in feelings of frustration and guilt as someone else takes on the task. Therefore, due to loss of the person's roles and physical health, feelings of losing the person can be experienced before actually losing the person.

Mental health professionals explore ways to reflect on the losses within anticipatory grief, to help manage and understand the emotions by providing the space to mourn losses, for both the patient and families. A mental health professional creates a safe environment where strategies can be made for redefining roles within the home and society (Hottensen, 2010). The charity Mesothelioma UK, Asbestos Support Groups, therapists and bereavement services have the potential to be this listening ear and offer support for anticipatory grief, facilitating patients and families through this conflict of holding on whilst letting go.

Attachment theory

Attachment is a key focus for therapists within the mesothelioma field. The psychologist John Bowlby explored the bonds people develop with one another and stated, "thus many of the most intense of all human emotions arise during the formation, the maintenance, the disruption, and the renewal of affectional bonds" (Bowlby, 1979). He emphasised that feelings of anxiety begin with a threat of loss or separation, with sorrow coming as a result of the actual loss. This can be complex depending on the individual's experience of attachment as a child which can bring up past trauma. It is common within mesothelioma to identify anxiety as a response to a loved one being taken away. "Bereave" stems from the same root as the word "rob" (Bowlby, 1980) and therefore what intensifies the disruption of the attachment bond further is the pain of a loved one's life being taken due to asbestos. It is therefore imperative to offer support from the point of diagnosis, to help the family as a whole navigate this disruption to their attachment bonds.

The importance of early-stage emotional support

The word bereavement is associated with support to those mourning post-death, however, many discussions have been based upon the necessity and benefits of support at an earlier stage (Holley & Mast, 2010; Parkes & Prigerson, 2010). Rando (1986) stated that when support is given after the death, there is nothing then that can alter the situation.

This knowledge helps inform what support should be offered to the patient and their family at the time of diagnosis/crisis, to share their worries and concerns, manage anxiety and recognise what is within their control. Rando suggested that when support is delayed until post-bereavement, we are trying to help a survivor when nothing can be done. However, when support is given in the pre-bereavement stage, it can have a profound and helpful influence post-death. As such, if bereavement services recognise the opportunity to create healthy endings in the pre-bereavement stage, they have the potential to improve the grieving process.

The stresses of family caregiving

Families often focus on the person with mesothelioma at the expense of their own wellbeing, whilst going through the physically and emotionally demanding "rollercoaster" of the disease (Prusak et al., 2021; Gibson et al., 2024). Families may have a perception that, whilst it is appropriate that care is focused on the person with mesothelioma, they have unaddressed support needs (Prusak et al., 2021). The distress and devastation of family experiences of diagnosis, treatment (if appropriate), witnessing symptoms and deterioration (Gibson et al., 2024) and then end of life can build into a lasting legacy of trauma (Lee et al., 2022).

Impact of end-of-life experiences

Family perceptions of whether a good death is achieved can have lasting impacts, both positive and negative. As noted previously in Chapter 9, evidence on whether people with mesothelioma are achieving a good death is sparse. The current limited evidence base highlights shortcomings in advanced planning with a lack of direct communication with families about the approach of end of life (Harrison et al., 2022); the potential for poor end-of-life care and negative impacts on families who witness poor symptom management (Nagamatsu et al., 2022); perceived inappropriate care (Harrison et al., 2022); and the distress and frustration of disjointed care (Harrison et al., 2022). The intensity of mesothelioma family end-of-life experiences can be magnified by witnessing a rapidity of decline and severe pain in their relatives. This can result in enduring emotional impacts (Gibson et al., 2014). In contrast families with positive end-of-life experiences can find comfort in knowing that their relative had been well cared for and they had done all they could. Experiences where families are able to fulfil their personal priorities mean that they are able to recount end of life in positive terms and this can be helpful in making sense of this difficult situation (Lee et al., 2022).

The role of families in end-of-life care can be very intense, and in particular if the death occurs at home. Families may undertake a physically and emotionally demanding role in organising care, administering medication and providing around-the-clock care (Gibson et al., 2024). This responsible role is combined with the emotional impact of trying to ensure a good death whilst working within health and social care systems which may not be sufficiently responsive to patient and family need to ensure optimal care. A recent study on family bereavement experiences in mesothelioma (SoS) found that families may be unprepared for the expectations of their caring role at end of life within the home (MURC, 2024). A lack of information about what support will be provided and knowledge around what to expect at end of life can mean that families may find themselves in stressful situations. In instances where difficult experiences were recounted, families often express satisfaction in knowing that their relative was able to die at home with family (especially if this was their wish). However, achieving this can come at a cost to families. In addition to this there can also be a lack of preparedness for the practicalities of what to do after a death (Harrison et al., 2022).

Bereavement experiences

Bereaved families can experience additional distress related to mesothelioma which impacts on experiences of grief and may lead to a need for counselling and support. A number of studies have highlighted how past experiences, such as a devastating and unexpected diagnosis of mesothelioma and providing care, were only processed in bereavement when families realised how difficult their experience had been (Prusak et al., 2021). Caring is an intensive experience which can leave a huge void when it is over, and at this point the past stresses may overwhelm families (Gibson et al., 2024). Families may also have neglected their own wellbeing in order to prioritise the care of their relative with mesothelioma, and then find in bereavement that they have reached a point of need (Ejegi-Memeh et al., 2024). An additional source of distress can arise from regret about the negative impact of treatments on mesothelioma patients. Warby et al.'s study

(2019) found that a quarter of carer participants (who were mostly bereaved) perceived that chemotherapy had done a lot of harm.

The injustice of asbestos exposure can impact on grief in different ways, with anger often experienced, due to the fact that mesothelioma deaths are preventable. Injustice can become a spur to become involved in collective campaigns for justice for mesothelioma, such as the Mesothelioma UK campaign "Don't let the dust settle". Participation in campaigns alongside other families impacted by mesothelioma can provide an opportunity to express and vent anger, and to find validation from collective experiences (Ejegi-Memeh et al., 2024).

Family experiences of supporting a relative with mesothelioma can engender an appreciation of the importance of family and friends and time spent together. A bereaved participant in a recent study (Ejegi-Memeh et al., 2024) described prioritising "making memories" with family in response to insights gained from mesothelioma of how life can be cut short. Support from healthcare professionals after the death of a loved one is particularly valued. In Ejegi-Memeh et al.'s study (2024) a bereaved participant recounted a chance meeting at a hospice with a healthcare professional whose impromptu hug was recollected with great appreciation. Bereaved families may wish to receive bereavement counselling and a post-death consultation with healthcare professionals (Warby et al., 2019)

Mental health support in bereavement

Bowlby (1979) has stated that those who avoid grieving are more likely to develop mental health problems. Mental health professionals can provide a space to consciously grieve. During the second stage of grief, after the death, the therapist takes into consideration the diagnosis experience, anticipatory grief, the loss of roles, witnessing of physical pain, end-of-life experiences, the breaking of affectional bonds and that mesothelioma is a preventable death. During this process the therapist can identify possible complicated grief, which may need to be resolved through trauma work. One mental health intervention that has had positive results is Eye Movement Desensitisation and Reprocessing (EMDR).

Implications for mental health practice

Bereavement services are an integral support within end-of-life care. They can take on many forms and be provided by a number of sectors, including Mesothelioma UK, hospices and specialist Asbestos Support Groups. Bereavement services mainly focus on the post-death experience; however, the anticipation of the loss is distressing and support at this time is invaluable. Grief is only one component of the mourning experience, other aspects include coping, psychosocial reorganisation, balancing conflicting demands, etc. (Rando, 2000), This can all be managed through appropriate support from bereavement services. Finally emotional support is essential from the mesothelioma diagnosis, continuing throughout the illness, end-of-life support and finally through bereavement counselling. The impact of mesothelioma is very individual and personal yet there is one commonality for all, asbestos.

Impact of coronial (or procurator fiscal) involvement

When someone with mesothelioma dies the coroner (or procurator fiscal (PF)) has to conduct an investigation. For some bereaved families coronial involvement underlines the difference in their experiences in comparison to usual practices around death.

The mesothelioma inquest procedure

One unusual feature of a mesothelioma diagnosis is knowing ahead of time that the patient's death will need to be referred to the coroner/PF. This gives professionals the opportunity to raise awareness of the coronial process in other professionals involved in the patient's care and the family, which can limit confusion and distress.

If a death is caused by, or is suspected to have been triggered by, an industrial cause the coroner is legally obliged to investigate. In most cases mesothelioma is caused by occupational asbestos exposure or via indirect exposure, for example, the wife of someone exposed at work (para-exposure). It is classed by the government as an industrial disease.

The coroner's role is to find out who the deceased is; and how, where and when they died. It does not mean there is a suspicion of any wrongdoing, and the coroner cannot apportion blame to individuals or organisations for the death. A coroner is usually a doctor or lawyer appointed by the local authority and each will have their own jurisdiction. There is no unified national coroner service in England and Wales.

When mesothelioma deaths occur in a hospital or hospice setting it is the responsibility of the medical professionals present to refer the death to the coroner. Mesothelioma deaths at home or in a care home setting are more complicated as a GP cannot issue a death certificate for deaths that need to be referred to a coroner.

Some community medical professionals are unaware that mesothelioma deaths should be referred to the coroner. Misunderstandings have occurred, causing confusion and distress for families. It is recommended that the patient's GP, district nursing team and palliative care team are made aware ahead of time that a referral to the coroner will be required.

In some local authorities it is the coroners' routine procedure to send the police to any deaths that occur at home. The police act as the coroners' representatives and complete an initial report which may include asking someone present to formally identify the deceased. Coroners in England and Wales have the autonomy to decide whether to send the police in these circumstances. It is recommended that you familiarise yourself with local procedures and find out if police attendance is routine in your area.

The coroner will assess the case and decide if a post-mortem is necessary for the investigation. Practice varies but, generally, if the patient's diagnosis was confirmed via biopsy in life the coroner will not usually carry out an examination.

In Scotland the Crown Office & Procurator Fiscal Service (COPFS) has responsibility to investigate all sudden, suspicious, accidental and unexplained deaths. It is a unified system and GPs can issue death certificates for mesothelioma if they have consulted with and been given consent to proceed by COPFS. Generally, if the patient's diagnosis was confirmed via biopsy in life the procurator fiscal will not carry out an examination. In Scotland the police are not routinely sent to mesothelioma deaths at home.

Impact on families of coronial involvement

The necessity for coronial involvement in mesothelioma deaths is an additional burden for families and can increase support needs (Guglielmucci et al., 2018; Sherborne et al., 2024a). Published literature highlights how the coronial processes (and for some, the ongoing legal action for compensation) adds to distress and requires families to focus on legal matters at a time of bereavement (Harrison et al., 2022). This lack of "closure" can interfere with bereavement processes (Clayson, 2003; Sherborne et al., 2024b). For some families the definitive diagnosis of mesothelioma is only received after a post-mortem (Sherborne et al., 2024a) and, in addition, the outcome of the inquest can impact on ongoing legal cases (Clayson, 2003). Whilst the resolution of legal cases for compensation after death can bring relief, there can be mixed emotions, including a perception that the compensation is "death money" (Sherborne et al., 2024b).

A recent study exploring UK family experiences of coronial involvement found both positive and negative impacts on families. A lack of information about the process was a factor in many of the negative impacts experienced, such as distress at finding out about the requirement for coronial involvement at a late stage (including either at, or after, the death). Some families struggled to understand why an inquest was required and found the concept of an inquest to be unfamiliar and bewildering. Bereaved partners in particular reported finding this stage of bereavement in parallel to the coronial process to be both lonely and isolating and some felt unsupported during this time. The concept of a post-mortem was emotionally demanding for some participants particularly if they considered it to be unnecessary as a definitive diagnosis had been achieved in life. Some participants found the concept of a post-mortem to be highly distressing as they did not wish their relatives to have to undergo this procedure when they had already suffered in life due to mesothelioma. The uncertainty of whether a post-mortem would take place was highly difficult, and participants valued being told at an early stage whether the post-mortem would take place. The coronial process was a barrier to families visiting the body of their loved one. In some instances, participants were distressed by not knowing where the body was and would have valued being informed of the location and when the body would be received by the undertaker. This presented a delay in observances around death which can be important to grieving families, such as visiting the body. In one instance the family were distressed to be told by the undertaker that the body had arrived in a poor condition from the morgue.

The main factor driving positive experiences of mesothelioma coronial involvement identified by the study was a family-centred empathetic approach. Examples included families feeling supported by coronial services who acknowledged and took account of their support needs, such as keeping families informed about what is happening and meeting families at the door when they attend the inquest. Participants who attended a face-to-face inquest at a court described feeling apprehensive and some found the formality of the process difficult. With hindsight they would have welcomed additional family-focused information to ease this experience, such as information about travel and parking, or knowing in advance that it would be helpful to take along a friend. Whilst some families in the study reported feeling a relief at the end of the inquest, for some this emphasised their loss, as the inquest had been a way of representing and supporting their loved one. A common legacy of family mesothelioma experiences is anger around the fact that their loved one's death was preventable. Families in this study expressed anger and talked about the injustice of asbestos exposure.

IMPLICATIONS FOR POLICY/PRACTICE

The evidence presented in this chapter highlights the needs of families whilst supporting their relatives with mesothelioma and during bereavement. This has implications and the following are recommendations for practice and policy.

- It is important that professionals have an awareness that families have support needs arising from their experiences from diagnosis onwards and that early-stage mesothelioma-specific support should be offered.
- Families may have increased support needs at different points within their loved one's illness that need to be acknowledged and addressed. Examples include, at diagnosis, end of active treatment, end of life of their loved one and during bereavement.
- Families need greater awareness of support services available to them, and in particular the availability of mesothelioma-specific support from, for example, Mesothelioma UK and the UK-wide network of Asbestos Support Groups (ASGs). Whilst the range of support services vary across ASGs, some provide tailored mental health support.
- Coroner services should ensure that the support needs of mesothelioma families going through the coronial process are addressed, such as through family-focused and sensitive communication and information sharing.
- Strategies are required to address the mental health impact of mesothelioma for families, for example, by increasing the awareness of the available support, such as the Mesothelioma UK Carers course.

CONCLUSION

Families' support needs can be unvoiced and unaddressed, and this increases the risk that families are burdened by the legacy of mesothelioma. The research data highlights family support needs across and beyond the mesothelioma disease trajectory and that legal processes may impact on bereavement. Care and support for families should be a central tenet for both professionals and support services. Strategies to increase the uptake of family support should address key barriers, such as a reluctance to seek help due to prioritising the needs of relatives with mesothelioma or a lack of awareness of how common difficult emotional impacts such as anger or loneliness are within mesothelioma families. An approach of repeatedly highlighting and offering support options for families would work towards signalling that their wellbeing is important, and also making them aware what support is available. The time after caring and during bereavement can be a time of greater need for mesothelioma families, and this should be a key time point when professionals and support services check in on families to find out if there are unaddressed needs.

REFERENCES

Bowlby, J. (1979). *The making and breaking of affectional bonds*. Oxon: Routledge.

Bowlby, J. (1980). *Attachment and loss: Volume 3. Loss, sadness and depression*. Middlesex: Penguin.

Clayson, H. (2003). Suffering in mesothelioma: Concepts and contexts. *Progress in Palliative Care*, 11(5), pp. 251–255. https://doi.org/10.1179/096992603322731143

Ejegi-Memeh, S., Sherborne, V., Mayland, C., Tod, A. & Taylor, B.H. (2024). Mental health and wellbeing in mesothelioma: A qualitative study exploring what helps the wellbeing of those living with this illness and their informal carers. *European Journal of Oncology Nursing*, 70, p. 102572.

Gibson, A.E., Ahmed, W., Longworth, L., Bennett, B., Daumont, M. & Darlison, L. (2024). Development of patient and caregiver conceptual models investigating the health-related quality of life impacts of malignant pleural mesothelioma. *Patient*, 17(5), pp. 551–563.

Goodreads (2016). *A grief observed quotes*. Available at: https://wwww.goodreads.com/quotes/649744-no-one-ever-told-me-that-grief-felt-so-like (Accessed: 25 March 2024)

Guglielmucci, F., Franzoi, I.G., Bonafede, M., Borgogno, F.V., Grosso, F. & Granieri, A. (2018). "The less I think about it, the better I feel": A thematic analysis of the subjective experience of malignant mesothelioma patients and their caregivers. *Frontiers in Psychology*, 9, p. 205.

Harrison, M., Darlison, L. & Gardiner, C. (2022). Understanding the experiences of end of life care for patients with mesothelioma from the perspective of bereaved family caregivers in the UK: A qualitative analysis. *Journal of Palliative Care*, 37(2), pp. 197–203.

Holley, C.K. & Mast, B.T. (2010). Predictors of anticipatory grief in dementia caregivers. *Clinical Gerontologist*, 33(3), pp. 223–236.

Hottensen, D. (2010). Anticipatory grief in patients with cancer. *Clinical Journal of Oncology Nursing*, 14(1).

Lee, J.T., Mittal, D.L., Warby, A., Kao, S., Dhillon, H.M. & Vardy, J.L. (2022). Dying of mesothelioma: A qualitative exploration of caregiver experiences. *European Journal of Cancer Care*, 31(5), p. e13627.

MURC (Mesothelioma UK Research Centre) (2024). *Supporting our Supporters (SoS): Improving the experience of family and caregivers of people with mesothelioma*. Available through: https://www.sheffield.ac.uk/murc/supporting-our-supporters (Accessed: 22 November 2024)

Nagamatsu, Y., Sakyo, Y., Barroga, E., Koni, R., Natori, Y. & Miyashita, M. (2022). Bereaved family members' perspectives of good death and quality of end-of-life care for malignant pleural mesothelioma patients: A cross-sectional study. *Journal of Clinical Medicine*, 11(9), p. 2541.

Parkes, C. M. & Prigerson, H.G. (2010). *Bereavement: Studies of grief in adult life* (4th ed.). Oxon: Routledge.

Prusak, A., van der Zwan, J.M., Aarts, M.J., Arber, A., Cornelissen, R., Burgers, S. & Duijts, S.F. (2021). The psychosocial impact of living with mesothelioma: Experiences and needs of patients and their carers regarding supportive care. *European Journal of Cancer Care*, 30(6), p. e13498.

Rando, T.A. (1986). *Loss and anticipatory grief*. Canada: Heath and Company.

Rando, T.A. (2000). *Clinical dimensions of anticipatory mourning: Theory and practice in working with the dying, their loved ones, and their caregivers*. USA: Malloy Lithographing.

Sherborne, V., Ejegi-Memeh, S., Tod, A.M., Taylor, B., Hargreaves, S. & Gardiner, C. (2024a). Living with mesothelioma: A systematic review of mental health and well-being impacts and interventions for patients and their informal carers. *BMJ Open*, 14(6), p. e075071.

Sherborne, V. Wood, E., Mayland, C.R., Gardiner, C., Lusted, C., Bibby, A., Tod, A., Taylor, B. & Ejegi-Memeh, S. (2024b). The mental health and well-being implications of a mesothelioma diagnosis: A mixed methods study. *European Journal of Oncology Nursing*, 70, p. 102545.

Taylor, B.H., Warnock, C. & Tod, A. (2019). Communication of a mesothelioma diagnosis: Developing recommendations to improve the patient experience. *BMJ Open Respiratory Research*, 6(1), p. e000413.

Warby, A., Dhillon, H.M., Kao, S. & Vardy, J.L. (2019). A survey of patient and caregiver experience with malignant pleural mesothelioma. *Supportive Care in Cancer*, 27, pp. 4675–4686.

Worden, J.W. (1983). *Grief counselling and grief therapy: A handbook for the mental health practitioner*. 2nd ed. London: Tavistock Publications Ltd.

Chapter 11

The role of primary care in mesothelioma

Emilie Couchman

OVERVIEW

In the UK, primary care is the gateway through which patients usually access healthcare services. People may alternatively self-refer to emergency services or privately to specialists. The terms *primary care* and *general practice* are often used interchangeably. However, primary care is the overarching sector of the healthcare system which includes general practice, pharmacy, dental, audiometry and optometry services; and general practice is the medical specialty aligned to primary care.

A general practice team may include general practitioners (GPs), nurses, physiotherapists, mental health practitioners, pharmacists, social prescribers and other allied health professionals (AHPs). The GP is not necessarily at the centre of a patient's healthcare experience nowadays, especially in the context of mesothelioma, where patients often engage with multiple clinicians from various disciplines in numerous settings. Further, given that people with mesothelioma often encounter healthcare professionals (HCPs) who are unfamiliar with mesothelioma, patients commonly feel the need to develop an expert level of knowledge about this condition. The role of the GP can thus be uncertain among both patients and professionals alike.

A commonly held perspective is that people both start and finish their mesothelioma journey with their GP. This is idealistic rather than realistic and does not ring true within current National Health Service (NHS) general practice. The increasingly fragmented, multidisciplinary healthcare system means that patients often struggle to maintain a relationship with an individual GP throughout their illness trajectory. For instance, if a GP refers a patient on a two-week-wait cancer pathway for suspected mesothelioma, they may not necessarily remain in touch throughout the treatment phase of the illness, transitioning seamlessly

DOI: 10.4324/9781032631318-11

into end-of-life care within this same clinician-patient relationship. It is beyond the scope of this chapter to discuss the impact of recent changes within the healthcare system on continuity of care, but it is becoming increasingly difficult to relate to the notion of the "family doctor" from "the good old days".

For patients who receive a diagnosis of mesothelioma, the implications can be catastrophic. With this incurable illness there are challenging symptoms; limited treatment options; legal implications given its status as an industrial disease; and a lack of understanding among the public and HCPs due to its rarity. The evidence relating to how people with mesothelioma experience primary healthcare will now be discussed, highlighting the need to define the role of general practice in alignment with the challenges specific to mesothelioma.

THE EVIDENCE

Ultimately, there is not enough evidence exploring the experiences of primary healthcare among people with mesothelioma and their close persons. There is no universal approach regarding the extent to which such individuals are involved with general practice. However, research exploring GP involvement in palliative cancer care has been categorised into three patterns: sequential; parallel; and shared care. In shared care, GPs are involved in a patient's cancer care; in parallel care, GPs are in contact with patients but are involved only with non-cancer issues; and in sequential care, patients are largely cared for by their oncologist after their diagnosis. (Norman et al., 2001) Further work is needed to identify characteristics relating to the patient, the clinician and the system that predict the degree of involvement an individual with mesothelioma may have with their GP and wider practice team.

Given the rarity of mesothelioma, it tends to be considered a disease to be managed by specialists; GPs and AHPs can therefore feel sidelined. For instance, the sense of isolation that patients may feel when consulting with an HCP who has never experienced caring for someone with their condition can be significant (Couchman, 2023) and some patients may consider their Mesothelioma UK clinical nurse specialist (MCNS) better placed to meet their needs. Disengagement with general practice may be a consequence. Such experiences also often prompts individuals with the capacity to do so to learn as much about the condition and available treatment options as they can. As such, the traditional doctor-patient relationship between the GP and individual living with mesothelioma is altered, and the role of the GP is different. However, patients with a range of cancer diagnoses want GPs to be more involved in holistic cancer care (Meiklejohn et al., 2016).

Certain tangible roles of GPs and AHPs in caring for people living with mesothelioma have been identified in the existing literature. They will now be discussed in turn.

- Maintaining up-to-date knowledge of mesothelioma
- Managing comorbidity
- Supporting informal carers
- Palliative and end-of-life care
- Coordination of multidisciplinary and interdisciplinary care
- Recognition of the mesothelioma patient's role in primary care

Maintaining up-to-date knowledge of mesothelioma

Clinicians in primary care must have sufficient knowledge of mesothelioma to identify potential risk factors and symptoms; initiate a timely referral to specialist services to enable diagnosis; recognise the implications and severity of such a diagnosis; and support patients to manage symptoms, make decisions and plan future care. For rare cancers such as mesothelioma, the potential lack of confidence among non-specialists may hinder their engagement with patients.

As stated in the General Medical Council's "Duties of a Doctor", doctors must keep their "professional knowledge and skills up to date" (General Medical Council, 2023). Mesothelioma does feature on medical school curricula but is often discussed as an afterthought to lung cancer. Existing literature widely recognises the many challenges unique to those living with mesothelioma that are not relevant in the context of lung cancer. Until recently, support for mesothelioma was based on existing care infrastructures established for lung cancer patients which fail to recognise the different needs in mesothelioma. There is also obviously a risk that those with peritoneal or pericardial disease are unseen and their needs are unmet.

Asbestos is currently the only known cause, categorising mesothelioma as an industrial disease. Increasingly though, people may have been exposed to asbestos in the domestic setting, such as when undertaking building work in their home, washing the clothes of a relative who worked with asbestos fibres or using talcum powder (Gordon et al., 2014). There is also a growing body of evidence suggesting that certain genetic mutations result in an amplified vulnerability to the carcinogenic effects of asbestos (Pagliuca et al., 2021) (see Chapters 2 and 13). Clinicians must be aware of the changing occupational risk and public health context of mesothelioma to facilitate timely diagnosis. Unfortunately, the common stereotype that only retired male shipyard workers contract mesothelioma is increasingly incorrect. Patients are being diagnosed younger; more of whom are female. Certain professions, such as teachers, are unfortunately at increased risk of developing mesothelioma. This highlights the need for HCPs to take a detailed occupational and social history in patients presenting with symptoms suggestive of mesothelioma, whether they are male or female.

Clinicians in primary care must be aware of the various treatment pathways available to patients if they are to provide appropriate ongoing support. Treatment options (including surgery, chemotherapy, radiotherapy and immunotherapy) remain limited, and generally only prolong life by a few months (Lim et al., 2023). Immunotherapy has drastically changed the landscape of mesothelioma care, especially in the way that patients interact with the healthcare system. For example, if a patient is receiving immunotherapy, they may be reviewed by the specialist hospital day unit team every three weeks prior to receiving their treatment. This may negate their need for GP involvement during this period. This may impede an ongoing clinician-patient relationship through a patient's disease trajectory and ultimately hinder end-of-life care planning in the community. Depending on individual patient factors, immunotherapy is available on the NHS and through clinical trial participation. It both inspires hope of longer life expectancy, but also adds stress given the uncertainty of its clinical effect, postcode lottery, lack of uniform funding on the NHS and need to participate in clinical trials to potentially receive it (see Chapter 5).

Managing comorbidity

People with mesothelioma may have other coexistent health conditions, with which their GP team may well be involved. For example, a diagnosis of type 2 diabetes mellitus may require a patient to attend their GP practice on a frequent basis for monitoring. Some patients consider their GP to be redundant regarding the management of their mesothelioma, as they would instead seek help from their MCNS relating to this disease. Again, there is insufficient evidence regarding the extent to which the characteristics of patients and HCPs in general practice lead them to engage with a patient's holistic care or not.

Supporting informal carers

"Informal care is generally defined as the unpaid care provided to older and dependent persons by a person with whom they have a social relationship, such as a spouse, parent, child, other relative, neighbour, friend or other non-kin" (Broese van Groenou & De Boer, 2016). People have varying levels of support and advocacy from their social network. If they have at least one close person by their side, patients may navigate the healthcare system in ways that better meet their needs, and they may be more resilient when faced with challenges (see Chapter 10).

As stated by Dr Cicely Saunders, the founder of the modern hospice movement, "how people die remains in the memory of those who live on" (AZ Quotes, 2024). The physical, emotional, psychological, social and financial toll on caregivers for people with mesothelioma is known to be significant. The symptoms experienced by individuals with mesothelioma can be significantly traumatic; if a caregiver has witnessed a loved one struggling for breath, the impact of their death will be even more upsetting.

A 2019 study exploring the burden of caregiving among those supporting a person with mesothelioma highlighted that more support for caregivers is needed (Moore et al., 2023). Informal caregiving is integral to the social care delivery system in the UK. Such individuals are "hidden patients" and their needs are often not recognised or met by healthcare services. Supporting caregivers adequately undoubtedly benefits the system, by improving outcomes for them as patients and for the patients they care for (Moore et al., 2023). Policy documents advise social care staff to identify healthcare needs among informal caregivers and direct them to their GP, however, the specific resources and infrastructure required for such service provision are often inadequate or inappropriate. Practices must keep a "Carers Register", a list of patients who provide support to a friend or relative with a health condition, but the resulting outputs are neither uniform nor mandatory within NHS primary care (NHS England, 2019).

Palliative and end-of-life care

Mesothelioma has a poor prognosis, with a median survival of between 8 to 14 months. There are no existing curative treatment options and such patients therefore have palliative care needs from diagnosis (Harrison et al., 2021). Palliative care is a core part of general practice and involves the timely identification and management of symptoms and psychosocial concerns for people with any life-threatening condition, and those important to them. End-of-life care is a subset of palliative care provided to people nearing the end of life, the timeframe of which varies depending on factors such as diagnosis, disease trajectory and patient preference (NHS England, 2023). Given its debilitating physical symptoms such as breathlessness, pain and lethargy; associated psychosocial impact for patients and families; and the fact that disease progression is often rapid, palliative care can play an important role at all stages of the mesothelioma trajectory (see Chapter 9).

In the UK, the majority of palliative and end-of-life care in the community is provided by GPs and other members of the general practice team. As the population ages with increasingly complex health and social care needs, people with a broader range of conditions are likely to have such needs. However, the recently published *Major*

Conditions Strategy from the Department of Health & Social Care identified that just under 50% of all people dying in England receive palliative and end-of-life care, which suggests considerable unmet need (Department of Health & Social Care, 2023). Similarly, findings from the UK National Mesothelioma Experience Survey found that unfortunately around 60% of people who desired support with palliative and end-of-life care needs did not receive it (Darlison et al., 2014).

As previously discussed, contemporary general practice involves a diverse, multidisciplinary group of HCPs. GPs work alongside district nurses, care home staff, homecare providers and specialist palliative care services. The field of community palliative and end-of-life care therefore faces comparable challenges, as it adjusts to the increasingly multidisciplinary style of service provision. People who are approaching the end of life therefore typically access care across multiple settings and organisations. It is vital that this care is effectively coordinated, and it is often the role of primary care clinicians to facilitate this. However, a recent systematic review highlighted that poor communication between professionals hindered the delivery of palliative care by GPs (Carey et al., 2019). Further, uniformity across geographical regions of the UK is lacking in terms of skill and training levels among staff; degree of integration of MDTs; communication across the primary secondary care interface; and access to specialist palliative and end-of-life care services (Mitchell et al., 2021).

Due to the tendency for patients with mesothelioma to experience a specialist-led healthcare journey, there can be a delayed or complicated transition to community-based palliative and end-of-life care after specialist treatment options are exhausted. A lack of effective communication between primary, secondary and tertiary care services limits a GP's capacity to support patient engagement with community palliative and end-of-life care services. For example, individuals with mesothelioma may not be recognised as being eligible for pathways such as the Gold Standards Framework or be added to the practice's Palliative Care Register.

Coordination of multidisciplinary and interdisciplinary care

The notion of the "multidisciplinary team" (MDT) has subtly different connotations in general practice than in secondary and tertiary care settings. In general practice, an MDT is designed to address the widening range of needs in each population. However, in the specialised context of mesothelioma, MDT working involves HCPs working together to meet a patient's specific needs with regards to mesothelioma.

In 2019, the Royal College of General Practitioners (RCGP) published *Fit for the Future*, their vision for general practice in 2030 (RCGP, 2019). The college's sentiment that "expanding the MDT is crucial if general practice is to meet growing demand and deliver a wider range of services in the community" (RCGP, 2023) reflected the ambitions of the 2019 NHS Long Term Plan (NHS, 2019). The intent to expand the workforce was made clear in policy by introduction of the Additional Roles Reimbursement Scheme. With this scheme, the government stated its intent to improve access to general practice, through the recruitment of 26,000 additional staff including first-contact physiotherapists, social prescribers, paramedics and pharmacists (Baird et al., 2022).

The UK NHS has undergone significant change since its inception, leading to changes in practice structure, out of hours (OOH) services, information technology infrastructure and GP contracts, all of which influence its ability to provide cohesive, integrated care (Gillam, 2017; Tan & Mays, 2014; Hill, 2011). This resonates internationally, for example, the Canadian primary care context has a reducing overall number of GPs, who are increasingly working part-time, relocating frequently and withdrawing from hospital work (Norman et al., 2001; Jones, 2019). Studies suggest that a single individual assuming a coordination role for patient care across the entire healthcare system is unworkable. General practitioners are seemingly no longer able to view the whole patient pathway, and then also take responsibility for coordinating patient care across the entire healthcare system. There may be scope for an alternative individual to take on this huge task, for example, the emerging clinical navigator position (Dalsted et al., 2011). Similarly, patients and close persons often report that the support provided by MCNSs resonates with such a role, particularly given their liaison across the primary secondary care interface (Gardiner et al., 2022). Ultimately though, there is a lack of clarity regarding whether HCPs working within primary, secondary or tertiary care should assume leading responsibility for people with mesothelioma. Patients are often uncertain about where to turn for help, and their decision-making process is compromised by a lack of collaborative working across healthcare settings. This is not unique to the mesothelioma context, and studies exploring the needs of patients with other rare cancers have noted poor relations between generalist and specialist HCPs (see Chapter 4) (Taylor et al., 2022).

Recognition of the mesothelioma patient's role in primary care

Despite the emphasis on patient-centred healthcare in the UK and internationally, the active role of the patient (and of their social circle) remains underexplored and inadequately facilitated by professionals (Coulter, 2006). Multiple factors are known to affect a patient's ability or willingness to assume an active role in partnership with their healthcare professional. These are very much dependent on context but may include elements such as: demographic characteristics; illness severity; health literacy; and healthcare setting. A *"patient's perception of their role and status as subordinate to clinicians"* has been identified as a barrier to patient engagement (Doherty & Stavropoulou, 2012, p. 261). Such impediments could be lessened by educational and cultural shifts, advocating the partnership approach to healthcare among both patients and HCPs (WHO, 2016).

People living with mesothelioma, and those supporting them, are often forced to develop an expert level of knowledge about this condition. Support groups are a valuable resource to such patients, given the relatively small community with a tendency to share self-directed learning. Previous research shows the contradictory predicament that patients with rare diseases often find themselves in. Such patients must often take responsibility for developing their own knowledge of their illness, its management and the required navigation of the healthcare service (Budych et al., 2012). However, studies show that those living with severe, incurable illness often prefer HCPs to initiate and take charge of decision-making (Schildmann et al., 2013).

IMPLICATIONS FOR POLICY/PRACTICE

The role of general practice in supporting patients with mesothelioma is often overlooked, compared with the perceived demand for specialist services. Primary, secondary and tertiary services should work together to support people living with or affected by mesothelioma. Collaborative working relies on effective communication across healthcare settings and interdisciplinary boundaries, facilitated by functional and reliable information technology systems. In the increasingly complex healthcare system, there is a great need for coordination and continuity to ensure that patients are negotiating and engaging with services to their utmost advantage. If a GP is to successfully integrate and coordinate a patient's care, they must be recognised by colleagues and patients alike as a key member of a patient's healthcare experience. However, the individual GP is no longer necessarily the glue that binds a practice team together, rather the inner workings and systems of a practice must provide this same assurance and cohesion.

Given the increasingly multidisciplinary nature of the care provided to and experienced by people with mesothelioma, clinicians should ascertain who patients identify as their key healthcare professional. For example, patients may view their MCNS as their first port of call. Patients should be encouraged to articulate their choices regarding care provision. Rather than providing strict recommendations as to how GPs should be involved in the care of people with mesothelioma, we should seek to understand the roles of HCPs working alongside and around the GP, so we may position the GP in each patient's sphere of healthcare experience on an individual basis. For some patients, their GP may be largely redundant (except perhaps for transactional queries such as issuing repeat prescriptions) as their needs are met by other members of the healthcare team. For others, perhaps with a longstanding relationship with their GP that predates their mesothelioma diagnosis, they may consider their GP to be a fundamental source of support. It remains unclear as to exactly how HCPs and patients are affected by the shift from the "family doctor" to the GPs' increasingly "medical consultant" style role as they collaborate with and oversee the practice of AHPs within the MDT (Modin et al., 2010).

Palliative and end-of-life care is a fundamental part of primary healthcare and is highly relevant to mesothelioma (WHO, 2018). A rise in the proportion of community deaths in many countries during the Covid pandemic was noted, especially in women and those dying of cancer. Such studies illustrate the increased pressure that general practice is under and are useful to direct palliative and end-of-life care resource allocation, depending on changing needs and preferences among populations (Lopes et al., 2024; ONS, 2021). High-quality community-based palliative and end-of-life care (either generalist or specialist, depending on the specific needs of the individual patient) is clearly essential if we are to meet the growing need of caring for those who wish to die at home. It must be explicitly acknowledged that people who die in hospital or hospice settings will still, more than likely, spend a considerable amount of time at home before they die, and thus it is not just those dying at home who engage with and benefit from community palliative and end-of-life care services. A recent multicountry study explored the impact on health-related quality of life among patients with pleural mesothelioma and their caregivers. The authors found that the psychological needs of patients and their caregivers increase significantly as the patient nears the end of life, and into the bereavement period (Gibson et al., 2024). Such knowledge can support policy and practice to prioritise focus on important time points in a patient's healthcare experience.

REFERENCES

AZ Quotes (2024). *Cicely Saunders quotes*. Available at: https://www.azquotes.com/author/20332-Cicely_Saunders (Accessed: 8 July 2024)

Baird, B., et al. (2022). *Integrating additional roles into primary care networks*. The King's Fund.

Broese van Groenou, M. & de Boer, A. (2016). Providing informal care in a changing society. *European Journal of Ageing*, 13, pp. 271–279.

Budych, K., Helms, T.M. & Schultz, C. (2012). How do patients with rare diseases experience the medical encounter? Exploring role behavior and its impact on patient-physician interaction. *Health Policy*, 105, pp. 154–164.

Carey, M.L., et al. (2019). Systematic review of barriers and enablers to the delivery of palliative care by primary care practitioners. *Palliative Medicine*, 33, pp. 1131–1145.

Couchman, E. (2023). Repetition breeds contempt, not continuity. *British Journal of General Practice*, 73, pp. 170.

Coulter, A. (2006). *Engaging patients in their healthcare: How is the UK doing relative to other countries?* Oxford: Picker Institute Europe.

Dalsted, R.J., Guassora, A.D. & Thorsen, T. (2011). Danish general practitioners only play a minor role in the coordination of cancer treatment. *Danish Medical Bulletin*, 58, p. A4222.

Darlison, L., Mckinley, D. & Moore, S. (2014). Findings from the National Mesothelioma Experience Survey. *Cancer Nursing Practice*, 13, pp. 32–38.

Department of Health & Social Care (2023). *Major conditions strategy: Case for change and our strategic framework*. Department of Health & Social Care.

Doherty, C. & Stavropoulou, C. (2012). Patients' willingness and ability to participate actively in the reduction of clinical errors: A systematic literature review. *Social Science & Medicine*, 75, pp. 257–263.

Gardiner, C., Harrison, M., Hargreaves, S. & Taylor, B. (2022). Clinical nurse specialist role in providing generalist and specialist palliative care: A qualitative study of mesothelioma clinical nurse specialists. *Journal of Advanced Nursing*, 78, pp. 2973–2982.

General Medical Council (2023). *Good Medical Practice: The duties of a doctor registered with the General Medical Council*. General Medical Council.

Gibson, A.E.J., et al. (2024). Development of patient and caregiver conceptual models investigating the health-related quality of life impacts of malignant pleural mesothelioma. *The Patient: Patient-Centered Outcomes Research*, 17, pp. 551–563.

Gillam, S. (2017). The Family Doctor Charter: 50 years on. *British Journal of General Practice*, 67, pp. 227–228.

Gordon, R.E., Fitzgerald, S. & Millette, J. (2014). Asbestos in commercial cosmetic talcum powder as a cause of mesothelioma in women. *International Journal of Occupational and Environmental Health*, 20, pp. 318–332.

Harrison, M., et al. (2021). Understanding the palliative care needs and experiences of people with mesothelioma and their family carers: an integrative systematic review. *Palliative Medicine*, 35, pp. 1039–1051.

Hill, A. & Freeman, G. (2011). *Promoting continuity of care in general practice*. Royal College of General Practitioners.

Jones, H. (2019). Working as a doctor in Canada. *British Medical Journal*, 367, p. l6971.

Lim, E., et al. (2023). MARS 2: extended pleurectomy decortication and chemotherapy for pleural mesothelioma. *International Association for the Study of Lung Cancer 2023 World Conference on Lung Cancer*. Singapore

Lopes, S., et al. (2024). The rise of home death in the COVID-19 pandemic: A population-based study of death certificate data for adults from 32 countries, 2012–2021. *The Lancet: eClinicalMedicine*, 68.

Meiklejohn, J.A., et al. (2016). The role of the GP in follow-up cancer care: A systematic literature review. *Journal of Cancer Survivorship*, 10, 990–1011.

Mitchell, S., et al. (2021). Community end-of-life care during the COVID-19 pandemic: Findings of a UK primary care survey. *BJGP Open*, 5(4), BJGPO.2021.0095.

Modin, S., Törnkvist, L., Furhoff, A.-K. & Hylander, I. (2010). Family physicians' experiences when collaborating with district nurses in home care-based medical treatment. A grounded theory study. *BMC Family Practice*, 11, p. 82.

Moore, A., Bennett, B., Taylor-Stokes, G. & Daumont, M.J. (2023). Caregivers of patients with malignant pleural mesothelioma: Who provides care, what care do they provide and what burden do they experience? *Quality of Life Research*, 32, pp. 2587–2599.

NHS (2019). *The NHS Long Term Plan*. National Health Service.

NHS England (2019). *Supporting carers in general practice: A framework of quality markers*. NHS England.

NHS England (2023). *Palliative and end of life care*. NHS England.

Norman, A., Sisler, J., Hack, T. & Harlos, M. (2001). Family physicians and cancer care. *Palliative care patients' perspectives. Canadian Family Physician*, 47, pp. 2009–2012.

Office of National Statistics (ONS) (2021). *Deaths from all causes by place of death, England and Wales, deaths registered in 2020 and average for 2015 to 2019*. Office for National Statistics.

Pagliuca, F., et al. (2021). Inherited predisposition to malignant mesothelioma: germline BAP1 mutations and beyond. *European Review for Medical and Pharmacological Sciences*, 25, pp. 4236–4246.

RCGP (2019*). Fit for the Future: A new plan for GPs and their patients*. Royal College of General Practitioners.

RCGP (2023). *Representing you: Policy areas: Multi-disciplinary teams*. Royal College of General Practitioners. Available at: https://www.rcgp.org.uk/representing-you/policy-areas/multi-disciplinary-teams (Accessed: May 2025)

Schildmann, J., et al. (2013). "One also needs a bit of trust in the doctor": A qualitative interview study with pancreatic cancer patients about their perceptions and views on information and treatment decision-making. *Annals of Oncology*, 24, pp. 2444–2449.

Tan, S. & Mays, N. (2014). Impact of initiatives to improve access to, and choice of, primary and urgent care in England: A systematic review. *Health Policy*, 118, pp. 304–315.

Taylor, A.K., Kausar, A., Chang, D., et al. (2022). "You know where we are if you need us." The role of primary care in supporting patients following pancreaticoduodenectomy for cancer: A qualitative study. *BJGP Open*, 6.

WHO (2016). *Patient engagement: Technical series on safer primary care*. Geneva: World Health Organization.

WHO (2018). Why palliative care is an essential function of primary health care. *Global Conference on Primary Health Care*. Kazakhstan: World Health Organization.

Chapter 12

Mental health and mesothelioma

Virginia Sherborne and Stephanie Ejegi-Memeh

OVERVIEW

Chapter 12 provides an overview of the psychological impacts of mesothelioma on patients and their family carers. The unique cluster of factors relating to mesothelioma are summarised, including the shock of the diagnosis, the disease's terminal nature and long latency period, the uncertainty regarding disease trajectory, and the availability of and access to treatments and trials. It also discusses some of the ways people living with mesothelioma, both patients and carers, manage the disease's impact. These include professional interventions as well as self-management strategies. Strategies to counter the sense of injustice from asbestos exposure and subsequent diagnosis are also covered. The chapter concludes with recommendations for policy and practice, such as the need for ongoing mental health education for healthcare professionals, signposting to mental health services and the importance of online and in-person social spaces.

THE EVIDENCE

In this chapter, we draw primarily on evidence from the *Investigating the Mental health Implications of a mesothelioma diagNosis and developiNg resources to Optimise Wellbeing* study, known as MINNOW (Ejegi-Memeh et al., 2024; Sherborne et al., 2024). Because little was known about the psychological effects of mesothelioma, we carried out this research study at the University of Sheffield in the UK (2022–2023). MINNOW aimed to answer three questions:

1 How does mesothelioma impact on patients and informal carers' mental health and wellbeing (MHWB)?
2 What is the scale of mental health conditions in these patients and carers?
3 What current psychological interventions are they using, and which do they find most helpful?

DOI: 10.4324/9781032631318-12

We hoped the study would help improve the quality of life for those living with mesothelioma by informing healthcare professionals how to provide enhanced support. We designed MINNOW as a four-phase mixed-methods study. The phases were a review of the existing research literature; a survey of mesothelioma patients and their informal carers, exploring positive and negative aspects of participants' mental health and wellbeing; interviews with 10 patients and 11 carers; and collaboration with patients, carers and practitioners to co-produce resources and recommendations for clinical practice. In this chapter we draw on results from Phase 2, the survey, and Phase 3, the interviews.

Research has shown that living with an incurable cancer potentially brings physical, psychological, financial and social difficulties. This applies to informal carers as well as patients. This type of diagnosis, with its threat to life and likely feeling of powerlessness, contains elements that may lead to psychological trauma. When people living with cancer experience uncertainty, for example, around treatment or prognosis, their quality of life can be negatively impacted. Cancer patients who experience pain are much more likely to have anxiety and depression and to feel unhappy with their treatment (Hoon et al., 2021).

When someone receives a diagnosis of mesothelioma, all these factors will be in play because of its incurable and terminal nature. On top of these, however, there are further aspects creating a unique set of effects on mental health and wellbeing. There is often a huge time lag between getting exposed to asbestos and mesothelioma symptoms manifesting. Pinpointing a definitive diagnosis can be challenging. Patients sometimes endure long waits and misdiagnoses. Receiving the diagnosis is usually a great shock for patients and carers (Sherborne et al., 2020). Along with the diagnosis, patients usually receive a prognosis, and for mesothelioma this can be very uncertain; survival times range from a few months to decades (Johnson et al., 2022). The progression of symptoms tends to be variable, with plateaux followed by sudden deterioration, and pain and cough can be challenging to control (Hoon et al., 2022; Slaven, 2023). The only known cause of mesothelioma is asbestos exposure, which has often happened in someone's place of work. This brings potential for psychological issues, as the relationship with a previous employer is in the mix. A patient and their relatives may have been long aware they were at risk of asbestos-related disease. The question of exposure brings a legal aspect involving such things as inquests and compensation claims, with stressful processes often consuming precious final months of a patient's life, and even continuing after their death (Lond et al., 2022; Nagamatsu et al., 2022). Mesothelioma is a rare cancer, which even healthcare professionals may not be familiar with. Access to new treatments and clinical trials tends to be limited. Those diagnosed with the rarer peritoneal form may feel especially overlooked. Also, as peritoneal mesothelioma patients are more likely to be younger and female, fertility issues bring extra negative impact.

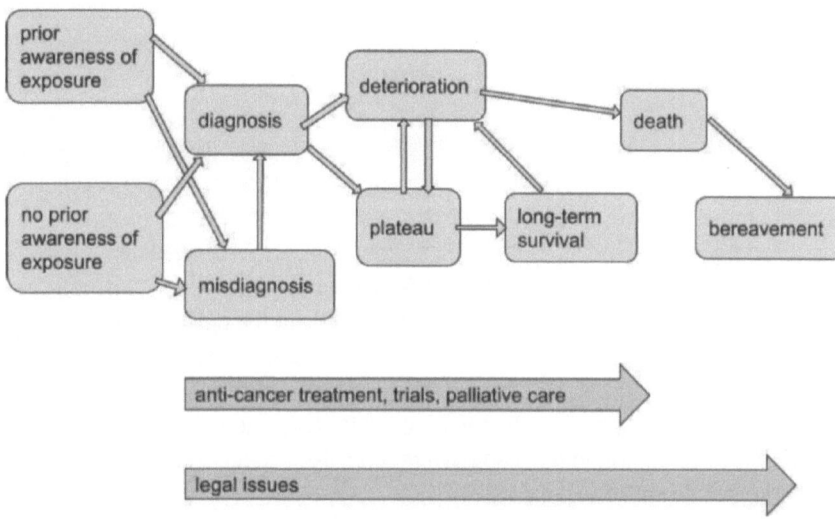

Figure 12.1 The complex and variable mesothelioma journey

The highly complex and variable nature of the mesothelioma journey can be seen in Figure 12.1. Psychological impacts can occur at any point in this journey. Carers may be similarly impacted to their loved ones, or their experience may be very different, which in itself can cause difficulties within families and relationships (Sherborne et al., 2020).

Existing research showed mesothelioma patients and carers experience a range of difficult emotions, including anger, frustration, depression, guilt, isolation, helplessness and distress, alongside upsetting changes in their sense of identity (Sherborne et al., 2020). However, it is important to mention that evidence also shows patients and carers living with cancer, including mesothelioma, can experience positive effects during their illness journey. These include relationships feeling deeper; life seeming more meaningful and fulfilling; and experiencing posttraumatic growth (Nouzari et al., 2019; Walker et al., 2019).

MINNOW survey results

The MINNOW survey provided insight into the levels of mental health impacts experienced in mesothelioma. Ninety-six people responded to the survey with enough completed answers to be meaningful. Of these, 35 were patients, 47 were carers and 14 did not say. Seventy-six participants were female and 20 were male.

We found some results showing levels which are potentially clinically significant. (For a firm diagnosis, an interview with a clinician would be required.) In the

Anxiety and Depression section of the survey, 29 people (30.2%) scored at a clinical level of depression, and half the participants at a clinical level of anxiety. One third of participants scored 44 or more on the PTSD scale, suggesting a clinical level of PTSD.

In the Posttraumatic Stress section, participants were asked to identify which aspect of their experience of mesothelioma was the most stressful. Patients identified the worst aspects as being "scanxiety" (anxiety when waiting for scans/results); waiting for and receiving the diagnosis; and experiencing medical interventions. For carers, the most stressful things were the diagnosis; witnessing their loved one's pain and feeling helpless; and fearing/experiencing their death.

When we compared the scores in each section for carers (current and bereaved) and for patients, we found that carers were more likely to report worse depression and PTSD symptoms than patients.

The survey questions about Posttraumatic Growth revealed that 34 participants (35.4%) had experienced personal growth in one or more of these areas: relating to others; new possibilities; personal strength; spiritual change and appreciation of life.

MINNOW interview results

From the interviews we developed three themes concerning mesothelioma's MHWB impacts: "Prognosis", "Support from services" and "Social connections and communication". These show how sometimes the illness journey affected patients and carers differently.

Prognosis

Usually given at the same time as diagnosis, prognosis caused patients and carers high negative psychological impact. Participants described this as a traumatic "death sentence":

> *"It's like being on the Green Mile but you haven't got any chance of appeal."*
> Susan (Patient)

The wording that healthcare professionals (HCPs) used about prognosis had a massive impact. Sian (Patient) was encouraged when her consultant said:

> *"We don't know what your journey's going to be like, but we're going to be here to support you."*

Graham (Patient), however, wanting reassurance, was left feeling unsupported, expecting imminent death. Being given details of expected deterioration brought anxiety for many patients. They worried about pain, breathlessness and becoming a burden. Eventually, though, some made peace with the death sentence:

> *"Once I realised that I was scared to die, I then found I could actually get on with living. Because I'd voiced the fear."*
>
> Ann (Patient)

Unexpected transitions anywhere in the journey brought anxiety, with the prognosis suddenly foregrounded. Scanxiety regularly occurred, worsened by delays. When the chance for new treatments or trials disappeared, panic could result.

Our participants' examples of depression spanned a spectrum from transitory low mood to severe clinical depression. For example, carer Jim spent six months having inpatient psychiatric care straight after the diagnosis. Low mood could happen at any illness stage, with uncertainty arising if patients survived beyond the original prognosis:

> *"I've had the treatment…It's this reality now…I'm going to die. That's the truth, out loud, and it's hit me."*
>
> Ray (Patient)

The prognosis even pushed a few patients and carers to think of suicide. Patient Ann was horrified that her husband could not bear to live with his "survivor's guilt". Carer Serena felt severe stress when her husband aimed for an immediate death from an exercise-induced cardiac arrest, instead of waiting to die from mesothelioma.

Eight participants mentioned experiences aligning with Traumatic Stress Symptoms (TSS). These are psychological symptoms experienced after a trauma, e.g. flashbacks, nightmares, dissociation, avoidance, irritability, guilt and isolation. Participants experienced these being triggered at different points in the journey. Traumatic moments included witnessing the moment of a syringe-driver being put in (carer Debbie) and having recurring nightmares ahead of the death (carer Crystal). One younger patient, Sian, got PTSD after a consultant suddenly disclosed her short prognosis when discussing fertility issues.

Several patients and carers showed prognosis-related posttraumatic growth, e.g. not taking things for granted; cherishing loved ones; making the most of the present:

> *"This last 18 months of my life has been really good, probably better than it would have been without a disease, I mean, because I've done more and I've been more positive."*

Susan (Patient)

Support from services

Participants highlighted that whilst HCPs and carers tended to focus on the patient's MHWB support needs, carers' needs were also important. Busy carers initially ignored their own needs:

> *"They [HCPs] always asked after dad. They never really asked how you were…I've never ever thought about talking about how I was feeling."*

Serena (Carer)

Some carers only recognised after the patient died that their own MHWB needs were unmet (see Chapter 10). Hindsight allowed them to judge that family self-care required promoting much earlier in the journey. They also highlighted that providing better advice on managing compensation could aid mental wellbeing:

> *"It's like death money. That's how I view it. There's no enjoyment…That's stress in itself, what do I do with it, where do I put it?"*

Laura (Carer)

Social connections and communication

Participants highlighted social connections and good communication as essential for MHWB. Support groups, like those provided by Mesothelioma UK and Asbestos Support Groups, allowed connection with others who understood. Some participants, though, mentioned barriers to attending, such as not wanting to be reminded of future deterioration.

Carers often mentioned expectations around giving and receiving support in the family, which could go unmet. Carer Crystal felt that she pressured herself too much:

> *"I gave myself such bad depression and I ruined my whole year of maternity leave."*

Carers in work had varied experiences of employers' support: some encountered flexible kindness, others had expectations smashed. Two abandoned long-standing jobs due to experiencing disloyalty and unhelpful communication.

Some participants mentioned higher anxiety about exposure to toxic substances, and could be negatively impacted by raising awareness about asbestos injustice:

> *"It is a ticking time bomb…I have got to draw a line under it, or it could really affect my mental health."*

> Serena (Carer)

Posttraumatic growth was often mentioned by patients and carers in its "relating to others" aspect, tending to focus on enhanced communication. Positive changes included increased emotional openness, calmness and selflessness; and enhanced closeness to loved ones.

Some participants mentioned "new possibilities", including openness to new relationships, involvement in asbestos activism and prioritising their time.

> *"I try to fill every minute…I'll only do what I want to do…If I don't fancy doing something, I won't…I've made new friendships, I've done new things, I try everything. Yeah, and probably a sort of renewed, if you like, zest for life really because I know how precious it is and how quickly things can change."*

> Laura (Carer)

What do people do to manage their mental health and wellbeing?

We found that patients and carers living with mesothelioma reported doing a number of things to manage the MHWB impacts described above. These included utilising self-management strategies, professional support and more informal social support. There was also evidence to suggest that patients and carers required different types of support throughout the experience of living with mesothelioma.

MINNOW participants reported that finding joy in exercise, nature, laughter and having family and milestone events to look forward to were important to their MHWB. Distraction was also often discussed as a useful tool for coping at times when mental health became challenging. The connection between good physical health and MHWB was also noted by several participants.

> *"When I come back from my hour's cycle ride, for example, I'm ready to take on the day."*

> Susan (Patient)

These small but impactful ways of creating and maintaining good MHWB were essential in the lives of the MINNOW participants.

Enjoying and nurturing relationships with family and friends were other ways in which both patients and carers dealt with a diagnosis of mesothelioma. For some this involved just spending time with their loved ones and for others this involved seeking financial compensation to ensure benefit for their loved ones. Planning for the future like this also gave a sense of control, which was important to participants. Other ways to gain control were making practical adaptations and getting involved in clinical decision-making, e.g. about joining a trial. Some activities combined several MHWB-enhancing strategies. This particularly applied to interacting with nature in a positive way (known as ecotherapy). For example, going for a ride on an electric bicycle in the countryside with friends would involve most of the strategies mentioned above.

Professional support was also highly valued by many participants, when available. This included support from clinical nurse specialists and doctors, who played a key role in both the provision of support and signposting to relevant mental health professionals and services. Being "held in mind" by professionals really helped both patients and carers not to feel abandoned or left in limbo. Professionals could provide this by regularly checking in throughout the illness journey. Despite the value placed on MHWB support by patients and carers, issues around availability of appropriate MHWB services were often identified.

Asbestos Support Groups and legal professionals played a unique role in the lives of patients and carers living with mesothelioma. They improved the MHWB experience by alleviating financial and administrative burdens.

> Interviewer: *"How did it make you feel that she [Asbestos Support Group professional] was coming and doing all that [benefits paperwork]?"*
>
> Jim (Carer): *"Fantastic. Absolutely fantastic, because I wasn't fully well myself and the thought of going through a 45 page form with [wife], which would be quite hurtful to her, you know, some of the questions asked, I was just totally elated by this person."*

The social support provided by Asbestos Support Groups is particularly important for people living with this rare, industrial disease. The rarity of mesothelioma means that many people find it important to connect with others who understand the condition. Therefore, coffee mornings and support group meetings can provide a vital space for people living with mesothelioma to feel understood and to reduce potential feelings of loneliness.

Social media and online connections were another way for participants to connect and share their experiences with others in similar situations. Social media, e.g. Facebook groups, were an important source of information and support for mental wellbeing, particularly for those living with the even more rare peritoneal mesothelioma. Furthermore, social media platforms made some people feel cared for.

> *"Like, obviously it's only Facebook posts, but a lot of people like it, or they put a caring emoji, or they'll put a comment. You know what I mean? We're thinking of you. That kind of…just supportive, right?"*

Ray (Patient)

However, some participants reported the need to silence social media notifications due to frequent death notifications in order to protect their MHWB.

The industrial nature of mesothelioma means that there is a social justice element. The act of campaigning and taking legal action against companies that caused asbestos exposure can provide a space to both access compensation and to channel anger at the injustice of being exposed to mesothelioma.

> *"I went recently to a demonstration about this asbestos company called Cape…It was like sort of shouting therapy. I was really shouting, like 'Shame on Cape! Cape must pay!'…I came away just feeling really good, and expressed some of that anger. And being in a group of people with that same anger."*

Olivia (Carer)

As we discussed above, patients and carers can have complex feelings around seeking compensation but, for some, knowing that they can financially provide for their families after their death was perceived as positive.

IMPLICATIONS FOR POLICY/PRACTICE

MINNOW findings suggested several areas for future research. Scanxiety is a significant issue for mesothelioma patients. Research is needed to better understand this experience and its effects. Evidence also shows that psychological trauma affects patients and carers living with mesothelioma. Trauma effects were both negative (traumatic stress) and positive (posttraumatic growth). More research into these would inform the provision of helpful interventions. Furthermore, future research also needs to focus on the evaluation of mental health and wellbeing interventions for patients and informal carers living with mesothelioma, so that we can understand what works for whom and when. Going forward, research that also focuses on positive MHWB outcomes is important to ensure that professionals, patients and carers can explore what works well and why in regards to MHWB.

Enhanced training and education around MHWB is also required in several areas. The delivery of diagnosis is a key factor in MHWB impact for patients and carers, so better awareness and training is needed for healthcare professionals. Supporting healthcare professionals to better identify MHWB impacts for both patients and carers via education and the use of validated, bespoke assessment tools is required. Only recently has posttraumatic growth been discussed in relation to mesothelioma so this area in particular requires attention in training for healthcare professionals. People working in law firms and Asbestos Support Groups would also benefit from ongoing training about the MHWB impacts so they can signpost patients and families, and consider the relevance for financial compensation.

Professional and informal MHWB support is key for both patients and carers. There is a need for better signposting and access routes to mental health services for patients and carers. Enhanced understanding is needed as to how people living with mesothelioma can get better access to mental health and wellbeing interventions (especially trauma-informed counselling, where appropriate). The creation and maintenance of online and in-person informal spaces for people living with this rare cancer are important. It is here that those that need to can connect, share coping strategies and even thrive living with mesothelioma. Carers may need encouragement to look after their own MHWB from the very beginning of the illness journey. This may include support to access mental health services, bespoke online or in-person sessions for carers or encouraging carers to just take time for themselves. For professionals involved in the care of people living with mesothelioma, awareness that carers may need to be reminded to look after their own MHWB may be helpful.

In the media, there has been recent acknowledgement of the extent and danger of asbestos exposure in public buildings, including schools, hospitals, etc. (Taylor et al., 2023). There is growing anxiety and anger about the risk of asbestos exposure which requires attention from a government policy perspective.

In this chapter, we have detailed how a diagnosis of mesothelioma impacts on the mental health and wellbeing of people living with mesothelioma and their families.

We found people experienced high levels of depression, anxiety and posttraumatic stress but also posttraumatic growth. Anxiety around scans was the most stressful aspect of living with mesothelioma for patients. For carers, it was aspects around their loved one's death. We also explored strategies that individuals and their loved ones use to maintain their mental health and wellbeing. These included spending time in nature, spending time with family and friends, distraction, seeking help from professionals and campaigning. We ended by making suggestions for future research, practice and policy.

REFERENCES

Ejegi-Memeh, S., Sherborne, V., Mayland, C., Tod, A. & Taylor, B.H. (2024). Mental health and wellbeing in mesothelioma: A qualitative study exploring what helps the wellbeing of those living with this illness ad their informal carers. *European Journal of Oncology Nursing*, 70, p. 102572. https://doi.org/10.1016/j.ejon.2024.102572

Hoon, S.N., et al. (2021). Symptom burden and unmet needs in malignant pleural mesothelioma: Exploratory analyses from the RESPECT-Meso Study. *Journal of Palliative Care*, 36(2), pp. 113–120. https://doi.org/10.1177/0825859720948975

Johnson, M., Allmark, P. & Tod, A. (2022). Living beyond expectations: A qualitative study into the experience of long-term survivors with pleural mespthelioma and their carers. *BMJ Open Respiratory Research*, 9, p. e001252. https://doi.org/10.1136/bmjresp-2022-001252

Lond, B., Quincey, K., Apps, L., Darlison, L. & Williamson, I. (2022). The experience of living with mesothelioma: A meta-ethnographic review and synthesis of the qualitative literature. *Health Psychology*, 41(5), pp. 343–355. https://doi.org/10.1037/hea0001166

Nagamatsu, Y., Sakyo, Y., Barroga, E., Koni, R., Natori, Y. & Miyashita, M. (2022). Depression and complicated grief, and associated factors, of bereaved family members of patients who died of malignant pleural mesothelioma in Japan. *Journal of Clinical Medicine*, 11(12), p. 3380. https://doi.org/10.3390/jcm11123380.

Nouzari, R., Najafi, S.S. & Momennasab, M. (2019). Post-traumatic growth among family caregivers of cancer patients and its association with social support and hope. *International Journal of Community Based Nursing and Midwifery*, 7(4), pp. 319–328. https://doi.org/10.30476/IJCBNM.2019.73959.0

Sherborne, V., Seymour, J., Taylor, B. & Tod, A. (2020). What are the psychological effects of mesothelioma on patients and their carers? A scoping review. *Psycho-Oncology*, 29(10), pp. 1464–1473. https://doi.org/10.1002/pon.5454

Sherborne, V., Wood, E., Mayland, C.R., Gardiner, C., Lusted, C., Bibby, A., Tod, A., Taylor, B. & Ejegi-Memeh, S. (2024). The mental health and well-being implications of a mesothelioma diagnosis: A mixed methods study. *European Journal of Oncology Nursing*, 70, p. 102545. https://doi.org/10.1016/j.ejon.2024.102545

Slaven, K. (2023). CO-051 Cough and mesothelioma (CAM): Emerging themes from a qualitative study exploring the impact of cough on quality of life. Poster presented to: International Mesothelioma Interest Group Conference, Lille, 27 June 2023.

Taylor, B., Tod, A. & Allmark, P. (2023). The hidden danger of asbestos in UK schools: "I don't think they realise how much risk it poses to students". *The Conversation*. Available at: https://theconversation.com/the-hidden-danger-of-asbestos-in-uk-schools-i-dont-think-they-realise-how-much-risk-it-poses-to-students-203582 (Accessed: 30 April 2024)

Walker, S., Crist, J., Shea, K., Holland, S. & Cacchione, P. (2019). The lived experience of persons with malignant pleural mesothelioma in the United States. *Cancer Nursing*, 44(2), p. E90–E98. https://doi.org/10.1097/NCC.0000000000000770

Chapter 13

Financial implications

Sarah Thomas

OVERVIEW

Illness can be the trigger that means people are eligible for and need to claim benefits and financial support. In this chapter we review the situation from the perspective of people with mesothelioma. First, we will examine why being diagnosed with some acute illnesses like cancer can necessitate people to engage with the benefit system. We will then explore why there are particular pressures for people with mesothelioma when they are applying for welfare or financial support. This will identify some barriers to claiming benefits and how to access specialist support. We will then provide a brief overview of some of the types of benefits or payments people can access in the UK. The next section will summarise some populations where barriers are experienced or where specific processes are in place to make a claim, i.e. women and people in or veterans of the armed forces. This chapter focuses on UK systems and benefits. Benefit system, processes and entitlements changes regularly. The content of this chapter was correct at the time of going to press.

THE EVIDENCE

Due to the nature of this chapter much of the content is based on descriptions of the relevant benefits and systems, experiences of those working with them and selected evidence where appropriate.

Illness and the benefit system

A wide range of benefits and financial support is available in the UK, covering lots of different situations and circumstances, but it can be difficult to easily access information about entitlements and find support with the claiming process. In addition, people with mesothelioma are often exploring benefit entitlements

DOI: 10.4324/9781032631318-13

whilst having extensive healthcare appointments. Proactive welfare rights advice services, working closely with health and social care professionals, can assist with the practical demands that arise from dealing with mesothelioma and should be considered an important part of a holistic approach to treatment.

Approximately nine out of ten cancer patients' households experience loss of income as a direct result of cancer (Moffat et al., 2010). Increased costs or loss of income can arise from a variety of issues such as a reduction or total loss of employment income for the patient and/or carer, increased travel costs, increased heating costs, changing dietary needs and purchase of household aids, adaptations and personal services such as gardening, cleaning and caring.

Many people with mesothelioma are already retired by the time of diagnosis so they rarely suffer a loss of employment income, however, significant physical decline can be swift. This can mean the patient has significant and multiple expenses related to the illness in a short period of time. From employing a gardening service to fitting a stairlift, the patient may need to draw on their cash reserves (if they have any) quickly.

For those mesothelioma patients who are not retired it is unlikely they will be able to return to the workplace for any significant amount of time post-diagnosis, especially if they are commencing treatment. They may be entitled to sick pay via their employer but there will be limits on the amount of time this can be claimed.

If the patient has a partner who is in employment, then they are also highly likely to require significant amounts of time off and will suffer financial losses as a result.

Mesothelioma and benefits

Mesothelioma is unique, when compared to other diseases, due to the number of different benefits that patients are eligible to claim. Not only are they entitled to the usual long-term illness and disability benefits that most cancer patients can claim, but they can also claim industrial injuries benefits and access government lump sum payment schemes. Most people with mesothelioma will be eligible for significant benefit payments.

Often people with mesothelioma think they will not qualify for benefits because their income is too high. A means-tested benefit is a benefit or payment which you can only claim if your income and/or savings are under a certain level set by the government. The level varies depending on your personal circumstances. Most benefits that people with mesothelioma are eligible for are not means-tested, so it doesn't matter how much income and/or savings they may or may not have – they will still qualify for a payment.

Patients are usually surprised by the level of benefit entitlement they have. Industrial injuries benefits and government compensation for mesothelioma patients are not well publicised or discussed outside of asbestos support professional networks. Most people will have had no previous dealings with the benefits system other than claiming their state pension and they usually require some reassurance that they are indeed eligible for these payments.

People with mesothelioma are often overloaded with information in the weeks following a diagnosis. While it is important to offer a patient benefits and compensation advice as soon as possible after diagnosis they may not be willing or able to engage with advice straightaway. Some patients are practical and ready to discuss these matters without delay, but some may need a couple of weeks, or longer, to process their diagnosis first. If a patient initially declines benefits advice, they may change their mind in the future. Therefore, ongoing access to support and advice is important. However, some are so overwhelmed they don't pursue entitlements. Others delegate this to a family member.

With the help from a specialist advisor the application process does not have to be unduly onerous or stressful. Most patients qualify for their benefits to be fast-tracked, due to their diagnosis and prognosis, avoiding lengthy wait times or additional medical assessments. People are often surprised by how smooth the process is and how little they have to do to get the payments.

One of the negative aspects of benefit and compensation entitlement is that it can provoke difficult emotions for the patients and their immediate family. Some of the amounts involved are significant and patients have often commented that it feels like "blood money". Some older people can be overwhelmed that they, at this late stage of life, are in a financially secure position after many years of frugal living. Meanwhile others, who may not have fully appreciated the seriousness of their diagnosis, find it brings home the nature of the disease and its incurability. However, once some time has passed, most patients are grateful for the extra income and find it reassuring that they will not be in any financial distress at this difficult time.

What can someone with mesothelioma claim?

There are two main factors that affect what the person with mesothelioma can claim, whether they are over or under state pension age and where their exposure to asbestos took place.

Disability benefits

At the time of writing there are standard disability and/or ill health benefits which are age-related and not means-tested. These benefits are to help with the extra costs associated with a disability or a long-term illness. If the patient is likely to have less than 12 months to live their claim will be fast-tracked and the maximum payment awarded with no need for a medical assessment, therefore, most mesothelioma patients will qualify for these benefits which are not means-tested.

- Attendance Allowance – for people over state pension age.
- Personal Independence Payment (PIP) –for people under state pension age.
- Disability Living Allowance (DLA) – adults can no longer make a new claim to DLA, however, if the patient is already receiving this benefit they may be able to get their payment increased.

When a person is awarded one of these benefits, it grants them access to a range of "passported benefits" which are entitlements, concessions and discounts derived from their eligibility for the primary disability benefit.

The weekly maximum payment for these benefits is currently £108.55 (2024–2025) and normally raises in line with inflation each April. People under state pension age who have significant mobility issues will also be entitled to an additional £75.75 per week (2024–2025).

There is no mobility-related benefit available to people over state pension age. If someone was already receiving a mobility-related benefit before they reached state pension age, then they can carry it over with them but no new applications for a mobility-related benefit can be made once state pension age is reached. This includes applications to the Motability scheme which allows people with certain disabilities to lease a car, scooter or powered wheelchair.

Additionally, mesothelioma patients will usually qualify for a Blue Badge, a government-issued permit for parking in designated disabled parking spaces.

Scotland

At the time of writing Scotland has a partially devolved benefits system and is in the process of rolling out replacements for the standard disability benefits. It has already implemented Adult Disability Payment which replaces PIP for Scottish claimants. In the future it will replace Attendance Allowance with Pension Age Disability Payment. The payment structure and amount remain the same but there are some procedural differences. One key difference is that the definition of terminal illness in Scotland (in relation to benefit claims) is different from the rest of the UK. Scotland does not require a healthcare professional to determine life expectancy if a person has a "progressive disease from which death may reasonably be expected".

In practice this means Scotland has two systems running concurrently when it comes to welfare benefits and a Scottish mesothelioma patient is likely to be entitled to benefits from both the Scottish and the wider UK government. Until the roll out of new benefits is completed the situation will be complex and fluid therefore it is essential that Scottish patients are referred to a Scottish specialist advisor.

Industrial Injuries Disablement Benefit

Industrial Injuries Disablement Benefit (IIDB) is not age-related and not means-tested. If the person's exposure to asbestos occurred while they were at work or on an approved employment training scheme or course in the UK, they can make a claim for IIDB.

To successfully claim IIDB the patient will need to provide information about their employment history – like the information you would find on a CV. In practice this can be the most challenging aspect of the benefits application process for some people and getting specialist advice is essential.

When it comes to employment and asbestos exposure people with mesothelioma tend to fall into the following categories:

- They know exactly where, when and how they were exposed.
- They are initially unsure but after some questioning and time to reflect on their employment history, a likely exposure route becomes clear.
- They suffer from cognitive or communication issues that are severe enough to prevent them from giving a firsthand account of their employment history and/or asbestos exposure; however, partners and/or family members can provide some information about employment and exposure.

With specialist support information on the person's employment history can be obtained from government departments such as His Majesty's Revenue and Customs (HMRC) and former work colleagues to help compile a comprehensive employment history and exposure statement. In some complex cases a specialist solicitor may be the best person to assist in compiling the employment history.

Information contained in the IIDB application must be consistent with the information contained in the civil compensation case as defendants in a civil case can request copies of the person's benefit application forms to look for any discrepancies.

It can take several weeks or longer to gather the information required to submit an IIDB claim. A balance must be made between the risk of sending incomplete or incorrect information versus the desire to get the benefit in payment as quickly as possible.

A successful IIDB claim is unlikely when:

- Despite thorough investigations no employment-related source of asbestos exposure can be identified.
- The person was self-employed when the exposure occurred.
- The person was living and working overseas for a foreign employer when the exposure occurred.
- The person suffers from cognitive or communication issues that are severe enough to prevent them from giving a firsthand account of their employment history and/or asbestos exposure and no relevant information can be gained from family members or acquaintances.

Mesothelioma patients are automatically entitled to the highest rate of IIDB which is currently £221.50 per week (2024–2025) and usually rises in line with inflation each April. Although IIDB is not means-tested it can affect the payment of any means-tested benefits that the person currently claims so again specialist advice is recommended. People will usually also qualify for an initial 13-week backdated payment, which they will receive in a lump sum.

If a person is awarded IIDB they may also be eligible for Constant Attendance Allowance and Exceptionally Severe Disablement Allowance if they have substantial care needs.

Government lump sum payments

The government has two mesothelioma lump sum payment schemes. These one-off payments are age related and are not means-tested. The person can only claim from one of the two schemes and a specialist advisor will help the person decide which scheme is appropriate for them. The payments are the same for both schemes.

If the exposure to asbestos occurred in the UK, regardless of how or when it happened, they will be eligible for a payment. Even if a person has no idea how they were exposed to asbestos, as long as they have not spent any significant time living in another country, they will be eligible for a payment.

Payments range from £114,210, for people aged 37 and under, to £17,745, for peoples aged 77 and over (2024–2025). Payments usually increase each year in line with inflation.

Government benefits and lump sum payments are separate from any civil compensation (see Chapter 14) that might be awarded in a legal case although, if civil compensation is awarded, then any government lump sum payments already received must be repaid. In some cases, IIDB must also be repaid but only up to the date of the legal agreement. IIDB received after the date of the legal agreement does not need to be repaid. The person's solicitor will arrange the repayment to the government via a deduction from the civil compensation settlement.

Women and industrial injuries benefits

Many women with mesothelioma face additional challenges in accessing benefits and seeking compensation.

The Gendered Experience of Mesothelioma Study (GEMS) gained insight into the needs of men and women with mesothelioma. GEMS involved interviews with 13 men and 11 women living with mesothelioma (Ejegi-Memeh et al., 2021b) and analysis of data on 1177 clients from an Asbestos Support Group in the south and south-east of England (Senek et al., 2020).

The GEMS study found that:

- 11.6% of women clients did not receive IIDB compared to only 3% of men.
- It took longer for women to claim IIDB than men.
- Women were less likely to seek legal advice than men.

Women diagnosed with mesothelioma, especially if they are over pension age, may be told by the probable cause of her exposure to asbestos is para-occupational, such as a husband or father who worked firsthand with asbestos. GEMS found that high-risk occupations differed for men and women and there should not be a presumption that women's exposure to asbestos is always para-occupational. They may have been exposed to chronic low levels of asbestos in their own working environments such as schools, hospitals and offices. This highlights the importance of specialist advisors to assess the working environments as well as the occupational role for women.

If a person's only source of asbestos exposure is para-occupational, it means they cannot apply for IIDB and their opportunities to pursue a civil legal case will be severely restricted.

Posthumous benefits

If claims were not made during the lifetime of someone with mesothelioma there are still posthumous options.

IIDB can be claimed posthumously but the maximum amount awarded will be 13 weeks' worth, backdated from the date of death. A claim can be made on behalf of the deceased and will be paid to their estate.

If posthumous IIDB is awarded, then they may also be able to claim 13 weeks' worth of Constant Attendance Allowance if the deceased had substantial care needs during the relevant period.

Government lump sum payments can be claimed posthumously but at a lower "dependant" rate than the rate paid had the person claimed within their lifetime. There are only certain people who are classed as dependants when it comes to eligibility to claim but it does include spouses, civil partners and dependent children. The payment is made directly to the dependent.

Standard ill health and disability benefits cannot be claimed posthumously.

Specific populations

In this section the experiences of people in the Armed Forces and those of different genders are examined in relation to claiming benefits.

Armed Forces

For UK Armed Forces personnel and veterans there is an additional layer of options to consider if they were exposed to asbestos during their service. Legal action against the Ministry of Defence (MOD) is not usually possible but, following a lobbying campaign by asbestos victim and veterans' interests' groups, the choice to access either a tax-free lump sum payment or a weekly War Pension has been available since 2015.

The one-off lump sum is £140,000 and the War Pension amount is variable, depending on the veteran's service and personal circumstances. Due to the typical prognosis of mesothelioma most veterans opt for the lump sum payment, however, if the veteran has a spouse, it is important to consider whether claiming a War Pension would provide more financial security in the long term, as it would allow their spouse to claim a War Widow/er's Pension. If the veteran opts for the lump sum payment a spouse cannot claim a War Widow/er's Pension.

An Armed Forces claim must be made, in life, by the person. No posthumous awards can be made so it is critical that Armed Forces veterans diagnosed with late-stage mesothelioma are advised to seek specialist advice immediately. Mesothelioma UK provides specialist benefits advice for veterans.

A recent study of UK military veterans with mesothelioma (the MiMES study) indicated that the nature and range of UK military veterans' asbestos exposure is varied and not just limited to high-risk occupations (Ejegi-Memeh et al., 2021a). Some participants were aware they may have been exposed to asbestos, but others had no idea prior to diagnosis. This influenced their experiences of diagnosis. Participants' military background had a bearing on their coping strategies after diagnosis. The study highlighted the importance of help in accessing support systems and participants preferred support from professionals with knowledge or experience of the military (Ejegi-Memeh et al., 2021a).

Dual exposure

Some veterans may have also been exposed to asbestos while working as a civilian. This is known as "dual exposure". Dual exposure means the person may be entitled to benefits and compensation through both the Armed Forces and civilian routes. The person will need specialist advice to identify and consider which options are the most appropriate for their circumstances.

UK citizens living abroad

Often Mesothelioma UK and other Asbestos Support Groups will receive enquiries from UK citizens living abroad who have been diagnosed with mesothelioma. Often these people were exposed in the UK and moved abroad later in life.

Some benefits can be claimed internationally but it depends on the country of the person's residence and whether they have a reciprocal welfare benefit agreement with the UK. UK citizens living abroad will usually be seeking UK legal advice as well as benefits advice so a referral to the Asbestos Support group closest to the location of their UK asbestos exposure is the recommended course of action.

Carers

The benefits system does provide support to unpaid carers, however, the eligibility criteria can be restrictive. The main benefit that unpaid carers may be eligible for is Carer's Allowance (CA). In order to receive CA, the cared-for person must be in receipt of certain disability benefits and require at least 35 hours of care per week.

The carer can be in paid employment and claim CA, but they must not receive earnings more than a set weekly amount, which increases each April. The limit is usually the equivalent of 15 hours at National Minimum Wage. Claimants of CA can face stiff penalties if they do not report earnings over this limit so it's especially important that people who claim CA and work keep a close eye on their earnings.

If the cared-for person is receiving means tested benefits, such as Pension Credit, Universal Credit, Housing Benefit and/or Council Tax Support it is important to check if those benefits would be affected by someone claiming CA. The cared-for person may receive an additional amount in their benefit called a severe disability premium. If someone claims CA for caring for them their severe disability payment will stop. An experienced welfare benefits advisor will be able to check how a CA claim would affect the cared-for person's benefits.

Carers over state pension age

CA is an "overlapping" benefit with state pension. On paper, a claimant can legitimately be entitled to both benefits however they can only receive the higher of the two payments. In the vast majority of cases state pension will be the higher of the two payments, therefore, most people over state pension age will not be able to receive a CA payment, despite meeting the eligibility criteria.

If the claimant has reached state pension age and is also claiming Pension Credit, then their payments will increase if they are eligible for CA. Pension Credit is a means-tested benefit for people over state pension age and on a low income.

Working age carers

Working age carers who meet the eligibility criteria for CA will receive the full weekly payment, currently £81.90 per week.

If the carer also claims a means-tested benefit the CA is classed as income and deducted, however, a Carer's Premium or Carer Element will be added to the claim instead. In practice this means if someone is claiming a means-tested benefit and then claims CA, their means-tested benefit will decrease slightly but, with the addition of the Carer's Premium/Carer's Element and the CA payment itself, the claimant will be better off overall.

In addition to CA, working age carers can also apply for Carer's Credit. Carer's Credit is a National Insurance credit that helps with gaps in someone's National Insurance record. This option is beneficial for people who have had to take time off paid employment to provide care which otherwise might affect their ability to qualify for a state pension.

IMPLICATIONS FOR POLICY/PRACTICE

It is clear from the detail given here that benefits for people with mesothelioma is a specialised area of welfare benefits advice. It is important to:

- Challenge any patients' assumptions that they will not qualify due to income or savings.
- Be conscious of stereotypes when it comes to asbestos exposure, especially with female patients, and encourage all patients to seek welfare benefits advice.
- Refer or signpost the person to an advisor who is experienced in industrial injuries claims.
- Refer as soon as possible after diagnosis.

Specialist welfare benefits advice is available by:

- Contacting the nearest Mesothelioma UK clinical nurse specialist to the person with mesothelioma.
- Contacting Mesothelioma UK.
- Visiting the Asbestos Victims Support Group Forum website to locate the persons nearest specialist support group: https://asbestosforum.org.uk/get-advice/#2.

In the UK, specialist welfare benefits advisors will often offer home visits as well as phone appointments. They will identify which benefits the person is entitled to, complete much of the paperwork on the person's behalf and ensure they receive their benefits as quickly as possible.

Some of these benefits cannot be backdated and some can only be backdated for a limited time. Others have a time limit for claiming, running from the date the person received their diagnosis. People should therefore be referred for specialist advice as soon as possible after diagnosis. Some benefits and payments can be made posthumously but the options are limited, and the payments are lower than if the person claimed in their lifetime.

There is great value in benefit advisors working closely with clinical and legal teams to provide seamless holistic support through an intense period following diagnosis and treatment for mesothelioma.

Downloadable resources and leaflets to order on benefits for patients with Mesothelioma are available at: www.mesothelioma.uk.com/benefits-advice/.

There are significant differences between the welfare benefits systems in England and Wales, Scotland and Northern Ireland. It is essential that patients are referred to an appropriate specialist advisor in their own country of residence.

Changes can and do occur in the UK benefits system on a regular basis. The information provided in this chapter was correct at the time of print.

REFERENCES

Ejegi-Memeh, S., Darlison, L., Moylan, A., Tod, A., Sherborne, V., Warnock, C. & Taylor, B.H. (2021a). Living with mesothelioma: A qualitative study of the experiences of male military veterans in the UK. *European Journal of Oncology Nursing*. https://doi.org/10.1016/j. ejon.2020.101889

Ejegi-Memeh, S., Robertson, S., Taylor, B., Darlison, L. & Tod, A. (2021b). Gender and the experiences of living with mesothelioma: a thematic analysis. *European Journal of Oncology Nursing*. https://doi.org/10.1016/j.ejon.2021.101966

Moffat, S., Noble, E. & Exley, C. (2010). "Done more for me in a fortnight than anybody done in all me life." How welfare rights advice can help people with cancer. *BMC Health Services Research*, 10. https://doi.org/10.1186/1472-6963-10-259

Senek, M., et al. (2020). Mesothelioma: Exploring gender differences in time to diagnosis, seeking legal advice and occupational risk. *Cancer Nursing Practice*. https://doi. org/10.7748/cnp.2020.e1745

Chapter 14

Seeking compensation

Jennifer Seavor

OVERVIEW

People diagnosed with mesothelioma not only have to deal with their diagnosis and digest treatment information and advice, but also turn their minds to the financial and practical implications of the disease for themselves and their families.

People living with mesothelioma in the UK and other countries may be able to seek compensation through a legal claim against those responsible for exposing them to asbestos. Pursuing a legal claim also allows people to secure funding for bespoke medical treatment. However, people may be motivated to pursue a claim for additional reasons.

This chapter will consider the experience of making a compensation claim and what may deter people from pursuing a claim. It will explore the reasons people should be encouraged to do so.

In addition, the chapter will summarise the settings in which people may have been exposed to asbestos, the role of specialist solicitors in gathering the evidence needed to pursue a claim and the process and legal framework for doing so. There will also be a focus on practical information for patients, caregivers and medical professionals where common questions regarding making a legal claim will be answered.

Countries will differ enormously regarding legal processes and systems, making it impossible to cover all jurisdictions in one chapter. This chapter will therefore focus on claims pursued in England and Wales.

DOI: 10.4324/9781032631318-14

EVIDENCE

Decision-making

Financial impact of a diagnosis of mesothelioma

It is difficult to imagine how devastating it must be to be told you have mesothelioma, which is incurable. To then realise that it is a preventable cancer must make it incredibly difficult to come to terms with. Whilst first thoughts may be about treatment, concerns may then turn to the practical and financial implications of the diagnosis. People may start to worry how they will pay their mortgage/rent and bills. Older people with mesothelioma start to think about how their spouse will cope before and after their death. A person with mesothelioma may worry how they will cope financially or who will provide care for them as and when the illness progresses. They may be the carer for their spouse or other family members and wonder how they will provide that care when they become ill themselves, or how their family will cope after they are gone. When someone is diagnosed with mesothelioma and they ask about what financial support is available, they are often advised to contact a solicitor about making a claim.

Why people may not seek legal advice or pursue a claim for compensation

Despite these worries, we know from research that many diagnosed with mesothelioma do not seek legal advice, or if they do, decide not to pursue a claim. Some of the likely reasons include being wary of solicitors, loyalty to employers and concern about any costs (see Figure 14.1).

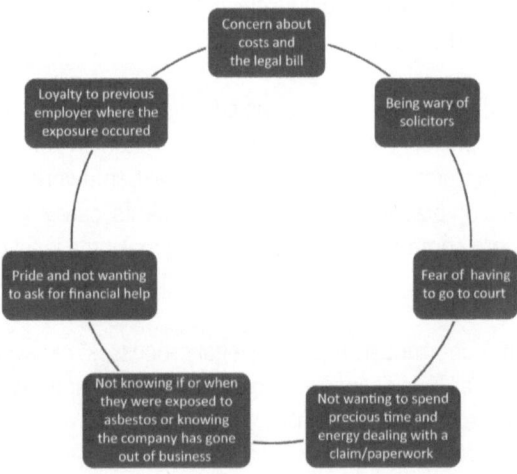

Figure 14.1 Factors hindering contact with a solicitor regarding a mesothelioma claim

Why people should make a claim

Despite having concerns, people with mesothelioma should be encouraged to seek initial legal advice from a specialist solicitor so an informed decision can be made. Whilst not all legal claims are successful, people with mesothelioma and/or their families rarely regret having tried. It should also be remembered that money may not be the prime motivation, there may be other reasons why pursuing a claim can be beneficial to the wellbeing of a person with mesothelioma or their family. Other motivations include the following: accessing non-NHS funded treatment, seeking justice, raising awareness and financial security for the family (see Figure 14.2).

Choosing a solicitor

It is vital that people seeking legal advice do so from a solicitor who specialises in mesothelioma claims. You would not instruct a solicitor who deals in divorce to do your conveyancing. Mesothelioma claims are very niche and for lawyers who do

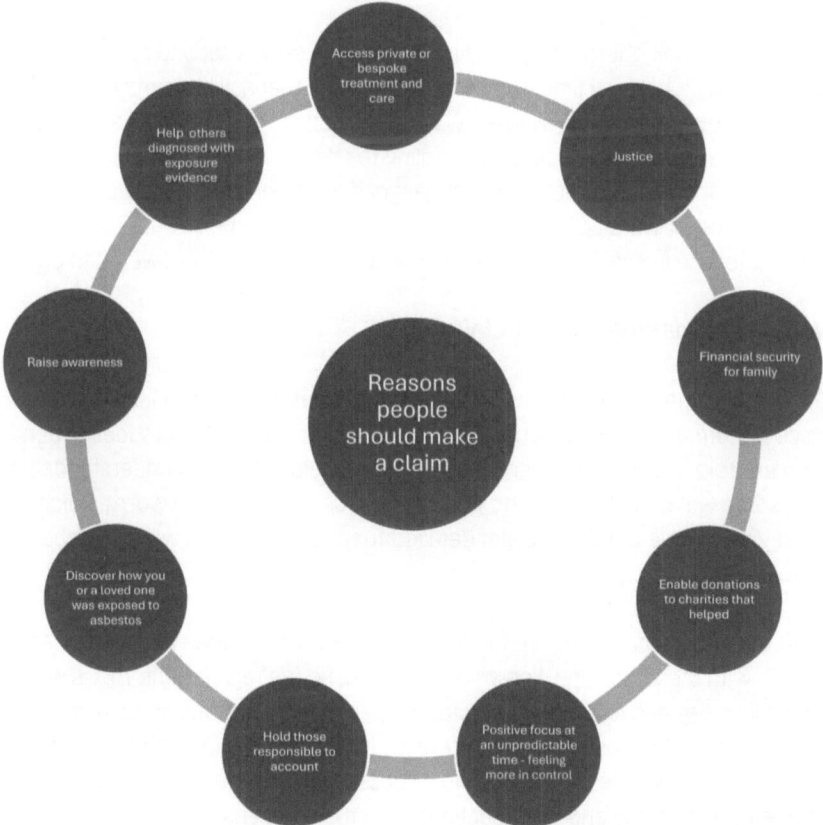

Figure 14.2 Reasons why people with mesothelioma pursue a legal claim

not practice in this area there can be many pitfalls. People should be signposted to a specialist firm. In the UK, the charity Mesothelioma UK has a panel of specialist firms, as do many regional Asbestos Support Groups.

Many specialist solicitors have had vast experience of being instructed by people with mesothelioma and are able to understand and assemble the evidence required to proceed with a claim in a timely manner. A specialist solicitor will utilise the fast-track mesothelioma section in the High Court and conduct the claim in a way which is more likely to lead to success.

It is vital that people have a good rapport with their appointed solicitor and feel confident in their abilities. There must be a mutual understanding of the person's aims. Not everyone simply wants to obtain the maximum compensation they are entitled to. For some an admission of liability is as important as the compensation itself, or an agreement ensuring they can access treatments not available on the NHS in the future should they need it.

People have the right to change their solicitor or to seek a second opinion from another solicitor, at any time. They should be aware that solicitors may have different views on the law, different ways of looking at their claims or different appetites for risk – some being more willing to take on more difficult claims. People may feel hopeless, frustrated and even angry if they feel they have not received good service, or were advised to no longer continue with the claim. People have nothing to lose in seeking a second opinion and should feel empowered to do so.

What will making a legal claim cost?

People with mesothelioma almost always ask what pursuing a claim is going to cost them and express concerns about having to pay solicitors fees. When they are told it won't cost them anything to make a claim, it is understandable that some will think that it is too good to be true. To add to the worry, solicitors must give people pursing a claim detailed funding paperwork which can be off-putting.

Most mesothelioma claims are funded with a contract between the solicitor and person with mesothelioma, known as a "no win, no fee" agreement. This is where the solicitor agrees to do legal work for the person who is stated to be responsible for payment of the costs incurred. However, in practice, the legal costs incurred will be recovered from the defendant(s) in a successful claim. There should be nothing for the person to pay and no deductions from the compensation agreed to put towards costs.

People often express concerns about what will happen if the claim cannot be taken forward after initial investigation, or if the claim is unsuccessful. The solicitor will not recover legal costs if the claim does not succeed. If the solicitor advises the person not to proceed with the claim perhaps through lack of evidence, or in the rare event that the case is heard in court and lost, no costs are payable to the person's own solicitor for the work they have done. The solicitor will usually arrange an insurance policy to cover any potential adverse costs which may be payable to the other side.

People should always be vigilant when entering into any agreement or contract, but if a specialist solicitor is instructed there should be no cause for concern.

What is the basis for a claim

How were you exposed to asbestos?

One of the first questions someone will be asked is whether they know how they were exposed to asbestos. For many this question is straightforward as they worked with asbestos and can name the company or companies they worked for. For others this question is much more difficult as they are less certain or perhaps have no idea of the circumstances in which they have come into contact with asbestos. Women in particular can find it hard to answer as most have not had traditional occupational exposure in the same way as men. People can also focus, sometimes incorrectly, on an incident or time in their lives where they think they were exposed and find it difficult to think beyond this, when in fact it is unlikely that this was exposure which caused their illness. An example of this is reporting possible recent exposures (within ten years of diagnosis) which medically will not be causative of their disease.

It is important, where possible, to take people through their entire life to consider all possible ways in which they may have been exposed to asbestos. This can be time-consuming, but it is vital. Many people actually enjoy telling their life story. This information will inform the best routes/defendants to pursue the claim against. Whilst it remains the case that occupational exposure is the most obvious, other forms of exposure should not be overlooked.

Someone may have been exposed occupationally, at work, or through para-occupational exposure through dust from family members' work clothes. Other routes of exposure include:

- Environmental exposure.
- As a bystander (close proximity to others using asbestos products).
- At school.

- From the fabric of buildings in disrepair or due to wear and tear or poor management of asbestos materials by occupiers of a building the person was working in or visiting.
- From contaminated talc products including body powder and make-up.

Of course, there may be occasions when someone is so unwell that a full history cannot be taken, and a solicitor has to work with brief information. In a posthumous case information may be given by family members who do not have much detail. All forms of exposure should still be considered where possible to ensure comprehensive advice is given and the claim is pursued in a way most likely to succeed.

Who to pursue the claim against?

People often believe that a claim is not possible because the company that was responsible for exposing them to asbestos is no longer trading. However, even if that is the case, most claims are dealt with by the company's historic insurers who can often be pursued directly. Where they are also defunct the Financial Services Compensation Scheme (FSCS) may step in.

What is the best route to pursue the claim?

Often people may have had multiple exposures, both occupational and other, and it is for the solicitor to advise tactically which company or organisation it is best to pursue. People often wonder how a claim can be pursued when it is not possible to prove 100% that a particular exposure caused the mesothelioma, and query which company or organisation should be sued when there may be several options. Special rules for mesothelioma mean that the law allows people to pursue just one defendant and recover full compensation from them, even if they have been exposed by multiple companies or organisations, or whilst self-employed too.

Multiple defendants/insurers may be pursued to achieve the best chance of success. However, sometimes as the claim goes on, and more information or evidence comes to light, or depending on the response of the defendant/insurers to the claim, defendants may be dropped. People can find this difficult as they may feel strongly that certain companies or organisations should be or should not be pursued. Solicitors are there to advise but people should always remember the solicitor acts for them and on their instructions. They should always feel able to discuss concerns with their solicitor or ask questions regarding the advice the solicitor is giving.

Building the case

Exploring the person's life

The first step will be for the solicitor to offer a face-to-face meeting – usually at a person's home so they do not need to travel. However, this meeting can be held in a hospital or hospice, the home of a family member or at the solicitor's office.

The information taken will be put into a witness statement. This is the most important piece of evidence in the claim. It is vital the contents are in the person's own words, to their recollections only, and that it is true and correct to the best of their memory, knowledge and belief.

Securing lifetime evidence in this way is an imperative and every effort should be made to do so, even if the person is not well. This is where the experience of a specialist solicitor is particularly important as they will know what the most pertinent questions to ask are. Evidence direct from the person with mesothelioma regarding the circumstances of their exposure can be crucial. Of course, people may not want the intrusion, and that has to be respected. However, where possible the meeting should go ahead.

Of course, claims can also be pursued posthumously and information, albeit perhaps more limited, can be taken from family members.

Record gathering and witness appeals

Depending on the information given, further investigation or evidence may be needed, in particular if there is uncertainty about exposure, dates or other facts. Specialist solicitors are again equipped to undertake these investigations, including seeking contemporaneous documents, researching in archives and local libraries and sending requests for assistance to other solicitors who may have pursued the same defendant(s) before.

Witness appeals are also often helpful. Adverts are placed in newspapers or on social media appealing for people to come forward to help if they worked at the same companies. People can find this daunting as it may mean revealing their name, making it public that they have developed mesothelioma and are pursuing a claim. However, it is often a vital element of investigations, particularly where the patient is unsure of their exposure. If the person or their family are really against this, anonymous appeals can be placed but where detailed evidence is still needed, ideally witnesses who worked directly with the person with mesothelioma need to be traced.

It is like a jigsaw piecing together information and evidence to build up the picture of what happened and prove the circumstances of exposure to asbestos.

Expert evidence

It is also necessary to obtain independent expert evidence to medically link the person's mesothelioma to their exposure, and to give an opinion as to their likely loss of life expectancy due to the disease. Experts have a duty to be objective and prepare their report for the court, not the person or their legal team. If someone has other health issues which could have impacted their life expectancy "but for" the mesothelioma, further medical evidence may be needed from experts in those specific fields. Evidence may also be needed for a spouse or partner to assess their own state of health. The report is prepared from the records, no examination is needed.

Legal framework

Burden of proof and establishing liability

Understandably most people diagnosed with mesothelioma have never pursued a legal claim before and have a limited understanding of what it will involve. The starting point is for the person to understand the burden of proof which in civil claims is the "balance of probabilities". Is it more likely than not that the person was exposed in the manner alleged, and that the exposure caused (i.e. materially increased the risk of them developing) mesothelioma?

Liability must be established. Compensation will not be recovered, or medical treatment paid for by the defendant(s) until liability is admitted, a court judgement in the person's favour obtained or settlement is negotiated with the defendant(s).

Court proceedings

The prospect of having to go to court and give evidence is for many one of the major worries about making a legal claim. However, in practice very few cases proceed to trial in court. Even if court proceedings are started usually cases will settle, or in some cases be discontinued, before a trial. Almost all hearings are dealt with by the lawyers and take place over the telephone. The person is not required to give evidence unless liability remains in dispute, or if liability is resolved but the amount of compensation to be paid cannot be agreed. If it is necessary for a person to give evidence this can sometimes be arranged in their own home or in an informal location close to their home, like at a hotel, rather than it being done in court.

Diffuse Mesothelioma Payment Scheme

The Diffuse Mesothelioma Payment Scheme (DMPS) was introduced in 2012 to compensate those who were exposed to asbestos at work but where the employers are no longer trading, and their insurers cannot be traced. Whilst welcome, it is not always sufficient as it only applies to exposure as an employee, it pays a fixed amount with no provision for medical treatment and the payments have not kept pace with inflation.

A solicitor can assist with a DMPS application at the appropriate time. It can be reasonable to submit an application early, whilst investigations are ongoing to trace insurers or perhaps whilst other routes of pursuing a civil claim are being explored.

Turner & Newall

Turner & Newall (T&N) were one of the largest asbestos product manufacturers in the country. They are now insolvent, but a scheme was set up to compensate those exposed to asbestos through their operations, not limited to those employed. Again, whilst not a legal claim in itself, a T&N application sometimes becomes part of the process and is something the solicitor will assist with.

Talc claims

Some people may be advised to contact a lawyer in America to pursue their claim in the USA on the basis of exposure from contaminated talc products such as body powder or make-up. Such claims are based on product liability which are rare in the UK. People will be asked to identify brands used and the frequency of use so lawyers can consider possible companies to pursue the claim against. Depending on where products were manufactured, it may be necessary for the person to have spent time in America in order to have the right to bring a claim in the jurisdiction, but this is not always necessary. People who bring a claim in this way usually have to be "deposed" or answer questions about their use of such products in front of a camera. The amount of compensation which can be recovered in the USA is significant as it is based on what a jury decides to award in each individual case. Multimillion pound verdicts have been reported.

Expatriates and exposure to asbestos in other countries

Jurisdictional issues may also need to be considered for people exposed to asbestos in other countries. Expatriates may have been exposed to asbestos in England/Wales then moved abroad at a later date. A claim can still be brought here but consideration should also be given as to whether it would be possible and even beneficial for the person to pursue a claim in the other country where they had exposure. Others may have used talc products and may have potentially been exposed to asbestos in that way and sometimes a claim in the US is appropriate.

Whilst specialist solicitors here cannot advise on the law in other countries, they can signpost people to take legal advice from lawyers in other jurisdictions. Even in the UK, the law in Scotland and Northern Ireland is different to that in England and Wales. It may be necessary for people to take additional advice in order to make an informed decision how to proceed with their claim.

Time limits

People have three years to make a claim. This is called limitation. This usually runs from the date they received their diagnosis but can on occasions be earlier. For example, if someone had symptoms they believed were due to asbestos exposure for some time before being diagnosed or they were diagnosed with another asbestos-related condition previously.

By the limitation date the claim has to have concluded, or court proceedings commenced by the issuing of a claim form at court. This stops the clock ticking and protects the person's position. Indeed, it can be a tactical decision to issue a claim form well before the three-year time limit, to secure an interim payment for the person/family or a court date against a defendant who is failing to engage or denying liability. Time is of the essence and sometimes commencing court proceedings is needed early to prevent delay.

Where someone has died from mesothelioma, their family or whoever is pursuing the claim on behalf of their estate usually have three years from their date of death to pursue a claim.

It is possible to bring claims outside the time limit, but this is dependent on the individual circumstances of a claim. The reasons for any delay should be explored and consideration given to the type of exposure, the likely defendant(s) and whether they would be prejudiced by the claim being brought later.

Time limits are something many are unaware of and it therefore falls to professionals involved in a person's diagnosis or care to raise the importance of seeking early advice. People should feel empowered to seek a second opinion about pursuing a late claim even if one solicitor tells them their claim is out of time. Sometimes the claim cannot be brought late or it is too risky to try to do so because of cost implications. However, people should be aware that if the three years has passed it does not automatically mean that there is no hope.

Also, there are different time limits in different jurisdictions, so it is advisable for people to seek advice without delay so as not to fall foul of deadlines or have missed opportunities. Likewise with the DMPS a claim must be submitted within three years of diagnosis and the time period does not reset on death as it does under civil law. It can be a minefield so the sooner someone takes advice the better.

Compensation

How much compensation will I receive?

Compensation can be a difficult subject for people to discuss as understandably they often may feel no amount of money can compensate them for what they may lose due to their mesothelioma – potentially many years of life. Whilst the law aims to put people in the position they would have been in had it not been for the defendant's breach of the law, or negligence, with mesothelioma that just isn't possible. Money cannot give people their life back. Talking in pounds and pence must seem very mercenary to some. However, other people take great comfort in knowing a claim will mean they and/or loved ones will be provided for.

Unfortunately, it is impossible to say at the outset how much compensation can be obtained as it is dependent on individual circumstances which need to be assessed. It is always in the tens of thousands of pounds, and more often than not in excess of £100,000. The compensation payable will be calculated on the following:

General damages

General damages are meant to compensate someone for the pain, suffering and loss of amenity caused by the illness. There are guidelines in place which give a bracket of compensation. Factors taken into account in assessing general damages include the person's age, the length of suffering, treatments sustained, side effects suffered and impact on life including whether the condition has prevented or restricted enjoyment of life, including hobbies. The bracket is currently between about £75,000 to £140,000.

Special damages

Special damages are any losses or expenses which the person has incurred, or may incur in the future as a direct result of their illness. The list below is not exhaustive but common special damages include:

- Income loss – loss of earnings and/or pensions.
- Care costs for the person, whether gratuitous, commercial or a mixture of both.
- Travel expenses.
- Services – things the person does or used to do that they will not be able to do as their illness progresses, or that will need replaced after their lifetime. Services can include cleaning, gardening, DIY, decorating, cooking, shopping, laundry, dog walking, childcare.
- Care for the person's spouse/partner/children.
- Aids and equipment such as a stairlift, adjustable bed, rise and recliner chair.
- Alterations to the home – grab rails, ramp, downstairs toilet, walk-in shower.
- Alternative accommodation – a person may live in an unsuitable property such as a high-rise building or flat where there isn't a lift and may need a more suitable property.
- Alternative therapies.
- Funeral expenses.
- Statutory bereavement damages.
- Hospice costs.
- Gifts.
- Any other loss directly flowing from the disease.

Non-NHS (private) treatment costs

Another important part of the compensation claim is the cost of non-NHS (private) or bespoke treatment costs, or an agreement with the company/companies or organisation(s) being pursued in the claim to fund treatment costs if and when such treatment is recommended by a person's oncologist at a later date. Advances in medicine through clinical trials and studies mean that new treatments may become available but not in an NHS setting in the time needed to benefit the person. Compensation can be sought to fund private treatment or an indemnity agreement put into place for the future if the person does not yet require treatment.

Settlement

Once a claim has been quantified the solicitor often seeks to settle the claim with the defendant(s) through negotiation. During this process offers may be made from both/all parties. People will need to consider with their solicitor the level of offer to make and/or whether to accept or reject offers made. Some can find this process stressful and worry if they reject an offer whether they are doing the right thing. However, the vast majority of claims conclude in this way, mostly to people's satisfaction, allowing the person or their family to get on with their lives.

IMPLICATIONS FOR POLICY/PRACTICE

Based on the above description of the compensation claims process a number of implications arise. First, it is a collective responsibility amongst professionals to encourage and empower people to seek legal advice, even where they do not know how they were exposed to asbestos, or their claim seems to be out of time.

Where necessary professionals should signpost people to a *specialist* solicitor. It is also important to understand the benefit of obtaining lifetime evidence where possible, recognising legal time limits, and encouraging people to act without delay.

Collaboration between medical professionals, specialist solicitors and charities improves patient experience. An open dialogue can also support patient decision-making between NHS treatment, clinical trials and private/bespoke treatments.

Chapter 15

Conclusion

Angela Tod, Clare Gardiner, Bethany Taylor and Liz Darlison

This book provides an overview of the experiences of people living with mesothelioma and those close to them. It seeks to provide a comprehensive view of what it is like to be affected by the illness and the challenges faced by those with mesothelioma, and their families. The content generates several key messages which are highlighted here as a conclusion.

Firstly, as a rare illness people with mesothelioma face a number of challenges shared with those experiencing other rare cancers and conditions, such as geographical isolation. With few people being diagnosed they're less likely to know, and get support from, other people with the condition. This increases the importance of services facilitating access to such support in terms of local, regional and national support services and groups. People with mesothelioma and other rare cancers also struggle at times to access specialist services as, for some, this means travelling long distances.

The physical and mental impacts of mesothelioma are profound, as indicated in Chapters 5 and 12. Specialist care and advice are therefore vital. This is increasingly important as new and emerging treatments are becoming available or evaluated in clinical trials. Most generalist health professionals, such as general practitioners, may not be aware of such advances and therefore not realise the urgency and importance of efficient referral for diagnosis and consideration for specialist care. New treatments and trials may not be suitable for everyone. Discussion with specialist staff is therefore even more important for people to understand the nuances of treatments and trials and the impact on their own lives and priorities. This book highlights how vital it is to communicate with people with mesothelioma with honesty and realism, whilst maintaining hope. This again indicates the importance of involving specialist services and personnel who are equipped to do this.

Mesothelioma is a complex condition creating several interrelated physical, emotional, legal and support needs. This book highlights the many aspects of

DOI: 10.4324/9781032631318-15

living with mesothelioma and the importance of providing personalised care that addresses the condition's complexity. The nurse specialist is often at the forefront of ensuring this happens, in partnership with other professionals and organisations. However, with current healthcare workforces under financial and recruitment pressure it is increasingly difficult to provide specialist nursing services without charitable support. This means people do not always have access to a specialist nurse in their area. In the UK, the Mesothelioma UK nursing network does provide a service to many, but not all, geographical areas. The charity is able to fill some gaps through services such as the telephone helpline. However, the fact that not all areas have a specialist nurse results in variation in care and difficulty for patients and families in accessing the care appropriate for their mesothelioma experience. Internationally, many countries do not have charities such as Mesothelioma UK facilitating access to support and care, making it more challenging to get the help required.

Providing tailored care is further challenged by the changing demographic of people being diagnosed with mesothelioma. There is increasing diversity in the population. Mesothelioma is not just occurring in people working directly with asbestos or in high-risk occupations, such as construction. More people working, living or being educated in buildings with asbestos in them are developing mesothelioma. This creates an urgent need to raise the awareness of atypical asbestos exposure amongst generic healthcare workers. They will then become more equipped to make timely referrals for diagnosis, treatment and care, thus avoiding some existing delays. There is also a demand for more awareness amongst the general public of the dangers of asbestos and what to do if they are concerned about how asbestos is managed in a building that they live, work or are being educated in.

A strong theme throughout this book is the impact of mesothelioma on families and close friends, as they face the multiple challenges associated with caring for someone with a life-limiting illness. Whilst the distress and emotional impact of mesothelioma can be immense for the person with the illness, family carers can experience an emotional burden that is different, but just as profound. The importance of caring for and supporting the family as well as the person with the disease emerges from the research presented in this book. In mesothelioma this support extends beyond health and social care and includes financial and legal support for families.

Another theme to emerge from this book is the importance of partnership working in providing care and support to people with mesothelioma. In the UK charities have an increasing role in providing, subsidising or underpinning the care provided by the NHS. This is evident in the UK through the role and scope of work conducted by Mesothelioma UK. However, other charitable and voluntary sector organisations also play a vital role, including Asbestos Support Groups. In addition, others are essential to successful partnership working including legal professionals. As identified here, the mesothelioma specialist nurse is often instrumental in ensuring input from any partners is included in a timely and patient-focused manner.

The focus of this book has been the experience of people in the UK with mesothelioma. Globally, rates of mesothelioma are stable, despite predictions of decreasing incidence. Whilst developed, more affluent nations sometimes struggle within their financial and service constraints to provide accessible care and support, the situation in low- and middle-income countries is of concern. For example, whilst India stopped mining asbestos in 1993, it continued to import the material. Much of their imported asbestos comes from Russia and Brazil (Jadhav & Gawde, 2019). This indicates the ongoing legacy of asbestos in these countries. Cases of mesothelioma are predicted to soar in India and other countries in future decades with an escalating demand for healthcare and treatments including, palliative and supportive care. The provision of tailored, appropriate and timely care is a concern, not just in the UK, but worldwide.

REFERENCE

Jadhav, A.V. & Gawde, N.C. (2019). Current asbestos exposure and future need for palliative care in India. *Indian Journal of Palliative Care*, 25(4), pp. 587–591. https://doi.org/10.4103/IJPC.IJPC_51_19

Index

Please note that page references to Figures will be in **bold**, while references to Tables are in *italics*.

abdominal symptoms of peritoneal mesothelioma 14, 34, 35, 61
ACCEND framework *see* Aspirant Cancer Career and Education Development (ACCEND) framework
access: to clinical trials 7, 15; to diagnosis and treatment xi, 2, 50–51; to experienced CNS/MCNS 15; inequalities in 50; to specialist knowledge 15; to support 16
Action Mesothelioma Day 27
activities of daily living 60
Advance Care Planning 58
AHPs *see* allied health professionals (AHPs)
allied health professionals (AHPs) 114, 115, 116, 122
analgesia/analgesic ladder 61
anti-angiogenesis agents 46
anticipatory grief 103–104, 107
antidepressants 66
antiemetics 64, 65
appetite, loss of 34, 48, 63, 66
Armed Forces 144–145
asbestos: banning/regulating in the UK (1999) 3, 8; bans in France and Germany 8; causing mesothelioma 2, 3, 4, 7, 8, 33, 35, 41, 102, 108, 126; continued use globally 16–17; expatriates and exposure in other countries 157–158; history of use and disease 8; how people were exposed to 153–154; injustice regarding effects of exposure 39, 107, 110, 125; latency

period for mesothelioma 2, 3, 9, 33, 103, 158; legacy in UK buildings 8–9; living near a factory 8; living with someone working with 8, 116; location of exposure 145; lung fibrosis 8; para-exposure 108; period of maximum importation and use of asbestos (1920–1970) 8; pre-1999 buildings 8; regulations to control 8; removal from buildings 17; by sector 7; stereotypes regarding exposure to 147; unawareness of exposure to 35, 39; use in steam-powered industries 8; *see also* healthcare sector, asbestos exposure; schools, asbestos exposure
Asbestos Support Groups (ASGs) 2, 5n1, 41, 82, 91, 107, 164; and bereavement 104, 107, 111; and financial implications of a diagnosis 139, 143, 145; and mental health 130, 132, 134; regional 152
ascites 13, 15, 53
ASGs *see* Asbestos Support Groups (ASGs)
Aspirant Cancer Career and Education Development (ACCEND) framework 22
aspiration, in MPE 51, 59
ATOMIC-Meso study 83
attachment theory 104–105
Attendance Allowance 4, 140
Australia 25

barriers to taking part in clinical trials: factors relating to healthcare professionals

(HCPs) 82–83; factors relating to mesothelioma patient 83–86; structural 81–82; *see also* clinical trials

benefits: Armed Forces 144–145; Attendance Allowance 4, 140; Carer's Allowance 146; Carer's Element 146, 147; Carer's Premium 146, 147; Constant Attendance Allowance 142; Disability Living Allowance 140; entitlement 139; Exceptionally Severe Disablement Allowance 142; government lump sum payments 142–143; illness and benefit system 137–138; Industrial Injuries Disablement Benefit 141–142; and mesothelioma 138–139; Pension Age Disability Payment 140; Personal Independence Payments 4, 140; posthumous 144; sick pay 138; specific populations 144–147; UK citizens living abroad 145; Universal Credit 146; what can be claimed 139–144; women and industrial injuries benefits 143–144; *see also* financial implications

benzodiazepines 60

bereavement experiences 25–26, 106–107

bevacizumab 46

biopsies 12, 34–35; results 35; video-assisted thoracic surgery 46

biphasic mesothelioma 12, 14

breathing exercises 60

breathlessness 3, 13, 118; in absence of pleural effusion 58; anaemia 58; non-pharmacological management 59–60; pharmacological management 60; pleural effusion causing 34, 58; pleural interventions 59; progressive 11, 58; respiratory infection 58; symptom management 58–60

British Thoracic Society (BTS) 13, 28, 65, 93

BTS *see* British Thoracic Society (BTS)

buildings, UK: asbestos in 8–9, 16–17, 35; pre-1999 8, 35

Cancer Alliance 25, 27, 28

carboplatin 46, 48

Carer's Allowance (CA) 146

chemotherapy options: doublet chemotherapy 83; side effects 48, 64; small survival benefit 50; standard of care 46

chest pain 34, 61

China, permitting of mining/use of asbestos 8

cisplatin 46, 48

Citizens' Advice Bureaux 41

clinical nurse specialist (CNS): in breast cancer care 23, 30; career development pathway 22; core member of multidisplinary team 23; development of role within cancer care 22–23; development of role within mesothelioma 5, 23–24; first roles in the UK 22; in lung cancer care 23, 30; and MDT 23, 30, 74; Mesothelioma UK 4–5; in palliative care 93; role in multidisciplinary and partnership working 21–32; strategies to enhance well-being 30–31; support following diagnosis 40–41; working at an enhanced or advanced level of practice 22; *see also* mesothelioma clinical nurse specialist (MCNS)

clinical research websites 83

clinical trials 3, 79–80; access to 7, 15, 50; aim of treatment, understanding 83; barriers/facilitators taking part in 81–86; discussing with nurses 82–83; evidence 80–88; experiences during 87–88; experiences following 88; expertise/trust in clinical team 85–86; HIT-MESO trial 82, 87; implications for policy and practice 88–89; obstacles 85; phases 80; practical issues impacting participation decisions 86; qualitative research studies 84, 85, 88; recruitment 87; role in mesothelioma 80; structural barriers 81–82; travel to hospital conducting 87; trial design 80–81; uncertainty of 85, 87

CNS *see* clinical nurse specialist (CNS)

Cognitive Behavioural Therapy (CBT) 60

colitis 64

colorectal specialty teams 35

combined chemotherapy treatment 46

Committee on Carcinogenicity of Chemicals in Food Consumer Products and the Environment, 2013 9

communicating a diagnosis 42, 43, 103, 128; evidence-based recommendations for practice 34; importance of good communication 33, 36; plain language

36–37; supportive environment 36; top
tips 42; *see also* diagnostic pathway
compensation, seeking 149–161; amount
159; basis for a claim 153–154; best route
to pursue claim 154; building the case
155–156; burden of proof/establishing
liability 156; burdensome process of 95;
costs of making a legal claim 152–153;
court proceedings 156; decision-making
150–152; Diffuse Mesothelioma Payment
Scheme 157; evidence 150–152; expert
evidence 156; exploring the patient's
life 155; financial impact of a diagnosis
150; general damages 159; how people
were exposed to asbestos 153–154;
implications for policy and practice 161;
legal framework 156–157; non-NHS
(private) treatment costs 160; reasons
for not seeking legal advice/pursuing
claim 150; record gathering and witness
appeals 155–156; settlement 160–161;
solicitor, choosing 151–152; special
damages 160; successful claims 37–38;
talc products 157; time limits 159–161;
Turner & Newall (T&N) 157; who to
pursue claim against 154; why claiming is
recommended 151; *see also* benefits
complex grief 95, 107
computed tomography (CT) scans 12, 13, 34
CONFIRM trial 46
Constant Attendance Allowance 142
constipation 34, 48, 57, 64; opioid-induced 65
COPFS *see* Crown Office & Procurator
Service (COPFS), Scotland
co-production 81, 97
coroner involvement 15, 38, 58, 70; in
England and Wales 109; impact of
108–110; investigations/inquiries 37,
92, 102, 108; reasons for 102; referral
to 108, 109; routine procedure 109; and
support for family 111; *see also* end-of-life
care; incurable and terminal condition,
mesothelioma as; inquest procedure
coronial (procurator fiscal) involvement
108–110
corticosteroids 64
cough 3, 34, 62–63; cough suppressants 63
court proceedings 156

COVID-19 pandemic 21, 28, 29; community
deaths 122
Crown Office & Procurator Service (COPFS),
Scotland 109
CT scans *see* computed tomography (CT)
scans
cytokines, pro-inflammatory 63

deaths from mesothelioma: during COVID-19
pandemic 122; at home 108, 109;
preventable 38, 39, 96, 102, 103, 107, 110,
150; referral to coroner 108, 109; support
following 107, 126; *see also* coroner
involvement; end-of-life care; inquest
procedure; palliative care; Procurator Fiscal,
Scotland; prognosis, in mesothelioma
decision-making: compensation, seeking
150–152; treatment experiences 49–50
Department of Health & Social Care 119
diagnostic delay 3, 14
diagnosis of mesothelioma 33–44; access to
2; biopsies 12, 34–35; and clinical trials 80;
communicating 33, 34, 42, 43, 103, 128;
as a process, not an event 40; evidence
34–41; family, effect on *see* family, effect
of a family-member's mesothelioma on;
financial and legal implications 37; first
steps 34; impact of receiving 38–39;
implications for policy and practice 41–43;
index of suspicion 10, 16, 17, 35; initial
differential diagnosis 36; length of process
34–36; mental health, impact on 38–39;
overloading with information following
139; personalising the diagnosis/
finding hope 39–40; pleural effusion,
breathlessness caused by 34; prognosis
38; rarity of 35; receiving of 36–38, 40;
retirement, in 103, 138; separation from
statistics 39; support, sources of 40–41;
uncertainty involved *see* uncertainty;
"watch and wait" recommendation 37, 45,
46; x-rays, ultrasound or CT scans 12, 34;
see also prognosis, in mesothelioma
diazepam 60
Diffuse Mesothelioma Payment Scheme
(DMPS) 157
digestive symptoms, in peritoneal
mesothelioma 34

Disability Living Allowance 140
domestic setting, exposure in 116
doublet chemotherapy 83
drug treatment *see* pharmacological treatment

Economic and Social Sciences Research Council (ESRC), Festival of Social Sciences 97
ecotherapy 132
education and asbestos exposure 9, 10, 17, 134
end-of-life care 95–96; defining 92; gaps in 95, 96–97; home setting 95; impact on family 105–106; and primary care 118–119; *see also* incurable and terminal condition, mesothelioma as; palliative care
EP/D *see* extended pleurectomy decortication (EP/D)
epithelioid mesothelioma 12, 14
EPP *see* extra-pleural pneumonectomy (EPP)
equipoise 81
European Respiratory Society 65
European Society for Medical Oncology 64
evidence: clinical trials 80–88; compensation, seeking 150–152; diagnostic pathway 34–41; financial implications 137–147; mental health and mesothelioma 125–136; palliative/end-of-life care 91–98; primary care, role in mesothelioma 115–121; risk factors for mesothelioma 8–16; role of MCNS 28; supportive care needs 70–76; symptom management 58–66; treatment experiences 45–53
Exceptionally Severe Disablement Allowance 142
experience-based research 4
expert evidence 156
extended pleurectomy decortication (EP/D) 47
extra-pleural pneumonectomy (EPP) 47
Eye Movement Desensitisation and Reprocessing (EMDR) 107

family, effect of a family-member's mesothelioma on 102–113; anticipatory grief 103–104, 107; attachment theory 104–105; bereavement experiences 106–107; clinical trials, attitudes to 85; diagnosis 103; early-stage emotional support, importance of 105; experiences across disease trajectory 103–105; follow-up care, experiences of 72; impact of coronial (or procurator fiscal) involvement 108–110; impact of end-of-life experiences 105–106; implications for policy and practice 111; lived experience 102, 104; magnitude of diagnosis, impact of 38–39; mental health considerations 39, 107; and mesothelioma as a preventable condition 103; and palliative/end-of-life care 96, 97–98; stresses of family caregiving 105; support for family 105, 107, 111
fatigue 3, 11, 13, 14, 34, 48; cancer-related 63; *see also* lethargy
financial implications 3–4, 137–148; advice services 41; dual exposure 145; evidence 137–147; policy and practice 147–148; *see also* benefits
Financial Services Compensation Scheme (FSCS) 154
follow-up care 70–71; delivery of 74–76; patient and family members' experiences of 72–74; views of people with mesothelioma on experiences of 73–74

gabapentin 61
GEMS *see* Gendered Experience of Mesothelioma Study (GEMS)
Gendered Experience of Mesothelioma Study (GEMS) 10, 17, 143
general damages 159
General Medical Council, "Duties of a Doctor" 116
general practitioners (GPs): multidisciplinary care 119; and primary care 114–116, 118; unlikely to initially diagnose mesothelioma 35; visits to 34
genetic mutations and vulnerability to mesothelioma 116
genomic medicine 27
Getting It Right First Time (GIRFT) programme 28
government lump sum payments 142–143
GPs *see* general practitioners (GPs)
gynaecology, referral to 35

HCPs *see* healthcare professionals (HCPs)

health and well-being, managing 131–133

Health Education England (HEE) 22

healthcare professionals (HCPs) 29, 37, 117; in A&E 34; access to 85; and clinical trials 79, 82–86, 88; communication of diagnosis 33, 34, 42, 43, 103, 128; and follow-up care 70, 71, 73, 74, 76; guidance for 41; hospital-based 10, 17, 57; infographic 97; key individuals, identifying 121; lack of experience regarding mesothelioma, where 42, 43, 114, 126; mental health education 125, 134; mesothelioma expertise, with 84; palliative/end-of-life care 91, 93, 94, 96–98; partnership with 120; on prognosis/life expectancy 38, 141; support following death 107, 126; training requirements 134

healthcare sector, asbestos exposure 7, 10, 17, 35, 134, 163

heavy industry 7, 10, 16

HEE *see* Health Education England (HEE)

HIPEC *see* hyperthermic intraperitoneal chemotherapy (HIPEC)

hospital-based staff 57; asbestos exposure 7, 10, 17, 35,134, 163

hot flushes 63

hypercapnia 60

hyperthermic intraperitoneal chemotherapy (HIPEC) 47

hypoxia 60

IASLC *see* International Association for the Study of Lung Cancer (IASLC) TNM classification of mesothelioma

IIDB *see* Industrial Injuries Disablement Benefit (IIDB)

immune-related adverse events (IRAEs) 49, 50, 53

immunohistochemistry tests 12

immunotherapy 3, 46, 48–49; "exceptional responders" 50; side effects 49, 64

income, loss of 138

incurable and terminal condition, mesothelioma as 1, 49, 65, 70, 79, 80, 126, 150; and the family 102, 103; and primary care 115, 121; *see also* coroner involvement; deaths from mesothelioma;

end-of-life care; inquest procedure; palliative care; Procurator Fiscal, Scotland

industrial disease, mesothelioma as 33, 102, 108, 115, 116, 132

industrial injuries benefits 139; and women 143–144

Industrial Injuries Disablement Benefit (IIDB) 3–4, 141–142, 144

indwelling plural catheter (IPC) 51–53, 59, 61

inflammatory cascades 64

informal carers 116, 117–118, 126; mental health and wellbeing 125, 133–134

inquest procedure 102, 108–109, 110, 126; *see also* incurable and terminal condition, mesothelioma as

intercostal nerves 61

interdisciplinary care 119–120

interferon-gamma 63

interleukin-6 63

International Association for the Study of Lung Cancer (IASLC) TNM classification of mesothelioma 13

International Mesothelioma Interest Group (iMig) 28

International Thoracic Oncology Forum (ITONF) 28

intestinal obstruction 15

intra and extra thoracic metastases 13

IPC *see* indwelling plural catheter (IPC)

ipilimumab 46

IRAEs *see* immune-related adverse events (IRAEs)

IRAMP study 84

ITONF *see* International Thoracic Oncology Forum (ITONF)

Japan 25

laparoscopy 46

laxatives 64

legal firms 41

lethargy 63, 118; *see also* fatigue

life expectancy 141; determining, in Scotland 141; extending 3, 45, 53, 117; health issues not mesothelioma-related affecting 156; impact of mesothelioma on 38, 65, 80, 156; *see also* deaths from mesothelioma; end-of-life care; diagnostic pathway; incurable and terminal condition, mesothelioma as; prognosis, in mesothelioma

lived experience of mesothelioma 1, 7–20; and AHPs 115, 116; challenges of living with 15–16; families living with legacy of 102, 104; and GPs 115, 116; implications for policy and practice 16–17; research rationale 2–4, 5; and role of the MCNS 94

long-term survivors 3, 45, 84; low number of 71, 72

lorazepam 60

lung cancer, distinguished from mesothelioma 11

lung fibrosis 8

Macmillan Cancer Support (MCS) 23

magnetic resonance imaging (MRI) 12

MAGs *see* Mesothelioma Asbestos Guidance Study (MAGs)

malignant pleural effusion (MPE): aspiration 51; breathlessness, causing 34, 58, 59; experience of management 52–53; long-term management 53; management of 51–52; non-expandable lung 59; and plural mesothelioma 11; recurrence 51; testing for 12; treatment experiences 51–52

Marie Curie (UK charity) 92

MARS2 trial 47; *see also* Mesothelioma and Radical Surgery 2 (MARS2) trial

MCNS *see* mesothelioma clinical nurse specialist (MCNS)

MCS *see* Macmillan Cancer Support (MCS)

MDTs *see* mesothelioma multidisciplinary teams (MDTs)

megestrol acetate 64

mental health and mesothelioma 125–136; evidence 125–136; impact of diagnosis 38–39; implications for policy and practice 133–135; management of health and well-being 131–133; mental health support for bereaved 107; MINNOW interview results 128–133; MINNOW survey results 127–133; prognosis of patient 128–130; social connections and communication 130–131; support from services 130

mental health and wellbeing (MHWB) 125, 128; of carers 134; enhanced training and education 134; and good physical health 131; importance of positive outcomes 134; management of 131, 132, 133; professional and informal support 134; services 132; social connections and communication 130

mesothelial cells 13

mesothelioma: and benefits *see* benefits; defining 1; deaths from see deaths from mesothelioma; diagnosis *see* diagnosis; as a disease 10–15; distinguished from other types of cancer 11, 13; experience-based research 4; failure to decline in the UK 3, 8; high rates in the UK 2, 7, 9–10; high symptom burden 57; increasing awareness of 16; inquest procedure 108–109; lack of public knowledge 28; multicystic 14; number of new cases per year 24; palliative care needs 91–93; pathology 7; pericardial 7, 10; peritoneal 7, 10, 11, 13–15; pleural 7, 10, 11–13, **11**; prevalence 1–2; as a preventable condition 38, 39, 96, 102, 103, 107, 110, 150; prognosis *see* prognosis, in mesothelioma; progressive nature of 12–13; rare nature of xi, xii, 2, 5, 10, 11, 15, 21, 34, 35, 37, 38, 41, 42, 53, 81, 96, 97, 116, 126, 132, 134, 162; regional centres 50; risk factors *see* risk factors for mesothelioma; seen as an industrial disease 33, 102, 108, 115, 116, 132; subtypes 12, 14; testicular 7, 10; third wave of 9–10; variation in care and treatment 15; women with 10, 17, 39, 48, 116, 126, 143; in younger people 9, 11, 39, 116, 126; *see also* asbestos; lived experience of mesothelioma

Mesothelioma and Radical Surgery 2 (MARS2) trial 47, 82, 84, 85, 87, 88

Mesothelioma Asbestos Guidance Study (MAGs) 10, 17

mesothelioma clinical nurse specialist (MCNS) 16, 21, 23, 24, 76, 83; ageing workforce 29; availability issues 85, 94; care coordination 26; and clinical trials 83; distinguished from other CNSs 24; evidence of value of role 28; implications for policy and practice 30–31; information resources/evaluation 26; key members of MDTs 26; Mesothelioma UK MCNS model regarded as gold standard 25, 28; and palliative care 94, 97; patient care 25–26, 30; and primary care 115; professional development 27; remit and role 25–28; service development/leadership 26–27; sustainability of posts 28; threats to role 21, 28–30; unique nature of role 23; working at an enhanced or advanced level of practice 24; see also clinical nurse specialist (CNS)

Mesothelioma Education Workers Study (MEWS) 10, 17

mesothelioma medical education 17

mesothelioma multidisciplinary teams (MDTs) 15, 16, 26, 43, 71; biopsy results discussed at meetings 35; CNS as core member 23; coordination of multidisciplinary and interdisciplinary care 119–120; integrated palliative care 94, 98; key workers within 67; living near 81; MCNSs key members of 26; mesothelioma clinical team 26; oncology 23; personalised treatment and follow-up by 71; requirement for concerning mesothelioma patients 66; and role of the CNS 23, 30, 74; specialist 15, 35; team meetings 35

Mesothelioma Service Framework 67

Mesothelioma Service Specifications 15

Mesothelioma UK 2, 4–5, 17, 41, 65, 71, 145; and claiming compensation 152; and clinical trials 82, 83; Clinical Trials app 89; and end-of-life care 91; and family support 104; free telephone support line 94; funding by 24; lack of resources 31; MCNS network 25; national nursing service 27; previously known as National MCS Mesothelioma Resource Centre 23; and professional development 27; support groups, locating 30

Mesothelioma UK Research Centre (MURC) 2, 4, 21; and palliative/end-of-life care 95–96, 97

mesothelium 1, 10

metastases: intra and extra thoracic 13; tract 48, 62

MEWS see Mesothelioma Education Workers Study (MEWS)

military veterans with mesothelioma (MiMES) study 145

Ministry of Defence (MOD) 144

MINNOW (Investigating the Mental health Implications of a mesothelioma diagNosis and developiNg resources to Optimise Wellbeing study) 125, 133; design of 126; as a four-phase mixed-methods study 126; interview results 128–133; and mental health 131, 132; and prognosis 128–130; survey results 127–133

mirtazapine 66

MPE see malignant pleural effusion (MPE)

MRI see magnetic resonance imaging (MRI)

multicystic mesothelioma 14

multidisciplinary care 119–120; see also mesothelioma multidisciplinary teams (MDTs)

MURC see Mesothelioma UK Research Centre (MURC)

National Cancer Registration and Analysis Service (NCRAS) 25

National Health Service see NHS (National Health Service)

National Lung Cancer Forum for Nurses 93

National MCS Mesothelioma Resource Centre (NMMRC) 23; see also Mesothelioma UK

National Mesothelioma Audit 2019 16

National Mesothelioma Audit 2020 13, 28

National Mesothelioma Framework 62

nausea 48, 57, 64, 65

neuropathic agents 61–62

neuropathic pain 61–62

neutropenia/neutropenic sepsis 48

NHS (National Health Service) 114; follow-up care 71; Long Term Plan (2019) 120; NHS Cancer Programme 25; NHS Wales 24

NHS Wales 24

NICE guidelines 28–29

nivolumab 46

NMMRC see National MCS Mesothelioma Resource Centre (NMMRC)

non-expandable lung 47, 52, 59, 63

non-pharmacological management: breathlessness 59–60; cough 63; psychological symptoms 65–66; systemic symptoms 63–64; *see also* pharmacological treatment; treatment experiences
nonsteroidal anti-inflammatory drugs (NSAIDs) 61, 64
Northern Ireland 24
NSAIDs *see* nonsteroidal anti-inflammatory drugs (NSAIDs)
nutritional supplements 63

ondansetron 64
opioids 60, 64; non-opioid responsive mesothelioma pain 62
oxygen therapy 60

pain, in mesothelioma 3, 11, 13, 118; abdominal 14, 34, 61; chest 34, 61; degree of severity 61; localised unilateral 62; neuropathic 61–62; pathophysiology of 96; uncontrolled 95
pain management 61–62
palliative care 91–101; access to 97; animation and infographic 97; care needs in mesothelioma 91–93; consultants 93; corticosteroids 64; early involvement of specialists 93; evidence 91–98; gaps in 96–97; healthcare professional infographic 97; implications for policy and practice 98–99; limited studies on, in the case of mesothelioma 93–94; MCNS roles 25; online event "Conversations about palliative care" (ESRC) 97–98; and primary care 118–119; providers in the case of mesothelioma 93–95; resources to support families and professionals 97–98; specialist services 57; as supportive cancer care 70; symptom control 57; *see also* end-of-life care
papillary mesothelial tumours 14
parietal peritoneum 13
partial pleurectomy (PP) 47
patient and public involvement (PPI) panel, MURC 97
PCC *see* percutaneous cervical cordotomy (PCC)

PCI *see* peritoneal cancer index (PCI)
pemetrexed 46, 48
Pension Age Disability Payment 140
percutaneous cervical cordotomy (PCC) 62
pericardial mesothelioma 7, 10
peripheral nerve blocks 62
peripheral neuropathy 48
peritoneal cancer index (PCI) 14
Peritoneal Malignancy Institute 27
peritoneal MCNS (PMCNS) 27
peritoneal mesothelioma 7, 10, 11, 13–15, **14**; abdominal symptoms 34, 35, 61; diagnostic period 35; incorrect initial diagnosis 36; lack of awareness of 43; limited research 72; rare nature of 133; surgical treatment 47
peritoneum 10, 13
Personal Independence Payments 4, 140
PET scans *see* positron emission tomography (PET) scans
pharmacological treatment: abdominal/gastrointestinal 64–65; breathlessness 60; cough 63; experience of 46; pain 61–62; psychological symptoms 66; systemic symptoms 64
pleura (lung lining) 1, 10, 53, 61; parietal 11, 47; thickened 11, 12–13, 59; visceral 11
pleural effusion *see* malignant pleural effusion (MPE)
pleural interventions 59
pleural mesothelioma 7, 10, 11–13, **11**; breathlessness due to fluid on the lungs 34; British Thoracic Society guideline 28; cough 62; existing knowledge based on 43; follow-up care 72; incorrect initial diagnosis 36; neuropathic pain 61–62; role of surgery in treatment of 47; staging of 13; surgical biopsies for 46–47; systemic treatment approaches 46
pleurodesis 46–47, 51, 59
PMCNS *see* peritoneal MCNS (PMCNS)
positron emission tomography (PET) scans 12
posthumous benefits 144
posttraumatic growth 127, 130, 133–135
posttraumatic stress disorder (PTSD) 92, 128, 129
PPI *see* patient and public involvement (PPI) panel, MURC

primary care, role in mesothelioma 114–124; comorbidity management 117; coordination of multidisciplinary and interdisciplinary care 119–120; evidence 115–121; implications for policy and practice 121–122; maintaining up-to-date knowledge 116–117; palliative and end-of-life care 118–119; recognition of mesothelioma patient's role in primary care 120–121

Procurator Fiscal, Scotland: impact of 108–110; investigations/inquiries 37, 102, 108; *see also* coroner involvement; deaths from mesothelioma; incurable and terminal condition, mesothelioma as; inquest procedure

prognosis, in mesothelioma 1, 38, 92; MINNOW study 128–130; posttraumatic growth, prognosis-related 130; survival beyond initial prognosis 129; uncertainty involved 38, 50, 65, 126; wording used by HCPs 128; *see also* diagnostic pathway; life expectancy

proton beam therapy 48, 82, 87

psychological intervention 125

"Pyramid of Care" model *75, 76*

qualitative research studies 48, 49; clinical trials 84, 85, 88

quality of life (QoL): and carers 94; and clinical trials 79, 80, 82, 87, 93; improving 45, 46, 49, 51–53, 70, 92, 126; maximising/optimising 53, 98; and palliative care 93; pharmacological treatment 64; reduced 15, 47; surgery affecting 59; symptom management 66, 67; symptoms of mesothelioma affecting 2, 57, 58, 61, 122; treatment affecting 50; uncertainty affecting 126

radiotherapy options 48; palliative 62

randomisation process 81

randomised controlled trials 46, 81, 87; multicentre 47, 93; *see also* clinical trials

rare cancers 6; charities 28; CNS role 21, 23, 30; contradictory predicament of those living with 121; mental health difficulties 15; mesothelioma as xi, xii, 2, 5, 10, 11, 15, 21, 34, 35, 37, 38, 41, 42, 53, 81, 96, 97, 116, 126, 132, 134, 162; as a percentage of all cancers 30; peritoneal mesothelioma 133; poor relations between generalist and specialist HCPs 120; progression of disease in 92; quality of life 15

RCGP *see* Royal College of General Practitioners (RCGP)

Receiving a Diagnosis of Mesothelioma (RADIO Meso) study 34, 40, 41

retirement, diagnosis in 103, 138

risk factors for mesothelioma 8–16; ageing buildings, exposure from 3; asbestos use *see* asbestos; construction, factory, mining and shipbuilding work 3, 7–10, 35, 163; heavy industry 7, 10, 16; limitations in data 9; new populations affected/changing demographic 3, 9, 43, 163; in schools 9, 10, 17, 134

Royal College of General Practitioners (RCGP), *Fit for the Future* 119–120

SACT *see* systemic anticancer therapy (SACT)

sarcomatoid mesothelioma 12, 14

'scanxiety' 72, 128, 129, 133

schools, asbestos exposure 9, 10, 17, 134

Scotland: Crown Office & Procurator Service 109; financial claims in 140–141; life expectancy, determining 141; Procurator Fiscal *see* Procurator Fiscal, Scotland; Scottish Mesothelioma Network 16, 24, 50

sertraline 66

settlement 160–161

side effects 37, 45, 46, 65, 66, 70; chemotherapy 48, 49; and clinical trials 80, 85, 87, 89; cough suppressants 63; gastrointestinal symptoms 64; general damages 159; immunotherapy 49, 64; megestrol acetate 64; new treatments 53; opioids 60; systemic 52

SPC *see* specialist palliative care (SPC)

special damages 160

specialist lung cancer teams 11

specialist palliative care (SPC) 93

staging of pleural mesothelioma 13

standards of care 15, 45–46

steam-powered industries, asbestos use as protection against high temperatures 8 support: access to 16; for bereaved 107; and coroner 111; for family 105, 107; mental health 134; sources, on diagnosis 40–41; *see also* Asbestos Support Groups (ASGs); supportive care needs

Supporting our Supporters (SoS) 104, 106

supportive care needs 69–78; evidence 70–76; follow-up care 70–71, 73–76; implications for policy and practice 76–77; other patients and families, connecting with 41; persons delivering 71–72; "Pyramid of Care" model 75, 76

surgical treatment 46–48; surgical pleurodesis 46–47

surveillance 70, 72, 74

sweating 34, 63

symptom management 57–68; abdominal/ gastrointestinal 64–65; breathlessness 58–60; cough 62–63; evidence 58–66; implications for policy and practice 66–67; interventions 62; pain 61–62; psychological symptoms 65–66; systemic symptoms 63–64; *see also* breathlessness; cough; fatigue; pain, in mesothelioma; weight loss

symptoms of mesothelioma: abdominal/ gastrointestinal 34, 35, 61; affecting quality of life 2, 57, 58, 61, 122; complexity of 92; gastrointestinal 64–65; managing *see* symptom management; psychological 65–66; systemic 63–64; Traumatic Stress Symptoms (TSS) 129; *see also* appetite, loss of; breathlessness; cough; fatigue; pain, in mesothelioma; weight loss

systemic anticancer therapy (SACT) 45, 46

talc pleurodesis 59

testicular mesothelioma 7, 10

thoracoscopy 12, 46, 51

tract metastases 48, 62

"trapped" lung *see* non-expandable lung

Traumatic Stress Symptoms (TSS) 129

treatment experiences 45–56; access to treatment 2, 7, 50–51; chemotherapy options 48; decision-making 49–50; drug treatment 46; evidence 45–53; immunotherapy 48–49; implications for policy and practice 53; limited treatment options for people with mesothelioma 79; malignant pleural effusion (MPE) 51–52; new emerging treatments 3; radiotherapy options 48; standard care 45–46; surgery 46–48; uncertainty as to 37, 49, 53, 81, 117, 126

tumour necrosis factor 63

Turner & Newall (T&N) 157

type 2 diabetes 117

ultrasound 12, 34

uncertainty: of clinical trials 85, 87; diagnostic period 35; exposure and dates 155; post-mortems 110; prognostic 38, 50, 65, 103, 126; progression of disease 92, 125; quality of life, impact on 126; on survival beyond initial prognosis 129; tests not detecting mesothelioma 35; as to treatment 37, 49, 53, 81, 117, 126

United States: development of CNS role in 22; and MCNS model 25; permitting of mining/use of asbestos 8

VCT *see* Virtual Clinical Trials (VCT)

video-assisted thoracic surgery (VATS) biopsy 46

Virtual Clinical Trials (VCT) 89

vomiting 57, 64, 65

Wales 24

weight loss 11, 13, 14, 63

witness appeals 155–156

women: deaths during COVID-19 pandemic 122; and industrial injuries benefits 137, 143; with mesothelioma 10, 17, 39, 48, 116, 126, 143

World Health Organisation (WTO): analgesic ladder 61; on palliative care 91–92

x-rays 12, 34

younger people with mesothelioma 9, 11, 39, 116, 126